The Family Guide
to Fighting Fat

The Family Guide to Fighting Fat

A Parent's Guide to Handling Obesity and Eating Issues

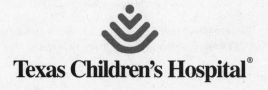

Texas Children's Hospital®

ST. MARTIN'S GRIFFIN ⚹ NEW YORK

www.stmartins.com

*A portion of Texas Children's Hospital's proceeds will be donated to the Center for
Childhood Obesity at Texas Children's Hospital.*

Library of Congress Cataloging-in-Publication Data

The family guide to fighting fat : a parent's guide to handling obesity and eating issues / Texas
Children's Hospital.—1st ed.
    p. cm.
Includes bibliographical references and index.
ISBN-13: 978-0-312-35786-3
ISBN-10: 0-312-35786-9
1. Obesity in children. 2. Diabetes in children—Prevention. 3. Eating disorders in children—
Prevention. 4. Children—Nutrition. I. Texas Children's Hospital.

RJ399.C6F3667 2007
618.92'398—dc22   2007013426

First Edition: October 2007

10 9 8 7 6 5 4 3 2 1

• • •

Note to the Reader

This book is for informational purposes only. It is not intended to take the place of medical advice from a trained medical professional. Readers are advised to consult a physician or other qualified health professional regarding diet and exercise or before acting on any of the information in this book. All patients' names have been changed to protect their privacy.

Contents

• • •

Acknowledgments

Obesity has become a major health issue facing families today. As clinicians, the authors know firsthand the struggles of families and the challenges children face growing up in an environment where food choices are too plentiful and exercise too limited. It is our hope that all who read this book will find some ideas and tools that will help them and their families be successful in achieving a healthy lifestyle.

The authors would like to thank the Texas Children's Hospital's executive team for their support of this project. The leadership for this project started at the top, with Mark Wallace, CEO, and Ralph Feigin, Physician-in-Chief, who heard the idea and created the environment to allow this book to be written. Tim Chafin, Vice President, early on helped to spearhead the design and development of the concept for the book. Myrtle Williams, Vice President, was also critical in the support of resources and excitement for the project.

The authors would also like to thank their many peers and fellow clinicians who in daily practice share ideas and tools, many of which are included in this book, to help make a difference in the management of childhood obesity. Dr. William Klish and Dr. Albert Hergenroeder were also invaluable for their content suggestions, medical expertise, and guidance as this book evolved.

A very special thank-you to our support staff, Stephen Steptoe and Brittan N. Clark, who helped with manuscript preparation.

Foreword

Over the past decade, the problem of obesity in children has received national and international attention. It has been the subject of numerous newspaper and magazine articles as well as television programs. The adverse consequences of obesity—including diabetes, hypertension, cirrhosis of the liver, sleep apnea, gallbladder disease, and the propensity for low self-esteem and depression—also have been documented extensively.

Obesity itself has contributed to an enormous increase in healthcare costs, while comorbidities of obesity not only burden individuals and families but also place a burden on the workplace and schools, causing inefficiency and absenteeism. A recent report from the Institute of Medicine of the National Academy of Sciences used the term "national epidemic" in describing this problem. The Centers for Disease Control and Prevention have called it "the single most important public health problem that faces the United States today" and have stated that this may be the first generation of children who fail to outlive their parents.

Thirty years ago, studies showed that only about 5 percent of children ages nineteen and under were overweight or obese. Today, more than 30 percent of children in the United States are classified as overweight, and roughly half of that group can be classified officially as obese. Considering that overweight children are 70 percent more likely than their normal-weight classmates to become overweight adults, we will be facing an even larger crisis in the years to come.

For these reasons, the publication of this book is most timely. It addresses all the issues that may be of interest to parents and their children with regard to the causes of obesity and the way parents and children can address or prevent this problem. Healthy habits and simple changes that families can make to promote weight loss are described in detail. Basic tips for adopting a healthy lifestyle, fun fitness options, food choices at home, school, and in restaurants, and advice concerning when it is appropriate for the family to call for help all are described. In addition, this book provides a customized plan applicable to each age group, from the first year of life through the prekindergarten child, the grade-school child, the middle-school child, and the child who is in high school. Finally, the book addresses what each of us can do within our home and community, as well as at the national level, to combat this enormous health crisis.

The book has been written by specialists in childcare, pediatricians, and subspecialists in pediatric medicine (gastroenterologists, dietitians, specialists in adolescent health, therapists, and others). The book is supported by the intellectual resources of Texas Children's Hospital and its pediatric faculty from the Baylor College of Medicine. It is also supported by the full resources of the Children's Nutrition Research Center, a program funded by the United States Department of Agriculture and operated in cooperation with Baylor College of Medicine and Texas Children's Hospital that has worked for almost three decades to define energy requirements, metabolism, and dietary requirements for pregnant women, newborn infants, young children, and adolescents. I enthusiastically recommend this authoritative resource for every family with children. If the recommendations contained herein are followed, we hope that future generations of children will outlive their parents.

—*Ralph D. Feigin, M.D., Physician-in-Chief, Texas Children's Hospital, and Chairman, Department of Pediatrics, Baylor College of Medicine*

· · ·

Introduction

The obesity epidemic is the number one public health crisis in the United States. Doctors, dietitians, and scientists have all explored many aspects of the problem characterized as being overweight or obese. The number of children who fall into these categories has nearly doubled in the last ten years. Unfortunately, no one has found a magic wand that will instantly make someone fit, but we have identified certain traits that help people find success along the road to better health.

Studies show that in order to change behaviors and habits, people must first believe they are capable of doing so. Your attitudes about healthy eating, exercise, and weight loss are your key to success because your motivation and commitment are a major influence on the success or failure of changing your eating, exercise, and food-buying habits.

Another part of that success is your family and your family's ability to work together to increase activity and improve eating choices. Studies show that a child's weight—which is directly affected by behaviors and habits—is more likely to change when all the family members adopt the same healthy routine. Consistent efforts by all family members support the child while also improving the entire family's health. Basically, healthy habits must become a way of life for your whole family.

Using This Book as Your Guide

The Family Guide to Fighting Fat is arranged to help you create a personalized plan for changing old habits and developing new, healthier ones.

The first step in making lifestyle changes is to develop an awareness of your family's current health status, eating behaviors, and activity levels. This awareness will help you make the changes you need to make to improve your family's health. The Family Assessment Tool below is designed to help you see and keep track of current patterns of behavior for you and your family. Take some time now to do the assessment. You will be using this information in Chapter 1 to help determine your family's readiness for change, the starting point for creating a personalized road map for success.

FAMILY ASSESSMENT TOOL

	Sun	Mon	Tues	Wed	Thurs	Fri	Sat	Total
1. How many hours per day does my child watch TV, play video or computer games?								
2. How many times per day do you drink soda or sweet drinks (including sports drinks)?								
3. How many hours do you exercise or have active playtime?								
4. How many times does the family eat out?								
5. How many times do you eat together as a family?								
6. How many servings of fruit and vegetables do you eat each day?								
7. Do you prepare meals and snacks that you plan for the day?								

Go to Appendix A for a full-size copy.

You will also want to examine which parenting and communication skills you will need to create change for improved health and weight loss. It will help to identify potential roadblocks on the path to success. Take time to consider all the outside factors that contribute to your family's ability to commit to a lifelong change. Think honestly about how committed you and various family members are to change.

Finally, you will need to set realistic goals and make health-conscious decisions for your family. The first chapter explains how to get started on the road to success, and each chapter continues to help you and your family set achievable goals.

Where Are You on the ROAD?

At the beginning of each chapter is a "ROAD" questionnaire. The acronym ROAD stands for

- **R**ole modeling, or the influence parents and family members have in shaping the food and exercise beliefs of a family.
- **O**rganizing and creating **o**pportunities for improved health behaviors, which may be as simple as a grocery list or planning a family outing.
- **A**vailability and **a**ccessibility of healthy food choices, because families cannot consume healthy foods if they are not available in the home or cannot be accessed easily by all family members.
- **D**ecisions must be made along the ROAD as you focus on changing behaviors that contribute to an increase in weight. These include setting goals, removing roadblocks, and taking detours when necessary.

The questions at the beginning of each chapter will assist you in evaluating your family's health, eating behaviors, and exercise habits, identifying roadblocks and barriers to success, and setting family goals. The second part of the book will help you do the same for your children, according to age group.

Think of a time when you have planned a family trip. You start with a map and get ready to go. With each self- or family quiz, you will be asked to score where your family is. Some families are truly just getting started on the ROAD to success. If your score is less than 4, you are beginning to look at the map and plotting strategies to improve your health. If you score between 4 and 8, your journey has begun, but be aware of the roadblocks in order to make it to your destination. If your score is between 9 and 12, you are well on the ROAD to better health, and your efforts should be directed toward staying the course and avoiding detours that may hinder you from reaching your destination.

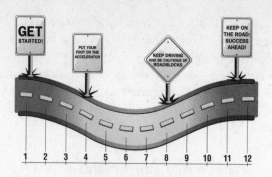

Putting It All Together

Chapter 1 provides you with background information about the principles of the ROAD and how to examine where you and your family are on the ROAD to success. It includes a process and tips for finding and writing simple, achievable goals.

At the end of the remaining chapters, you will be able to reexamine your habits in light of new information provided in that chapter. You can look back at the answers you marked on the questionnaire at the beginning of the chapter and consider ways to create change. These chapters also provide examples of goals that might be specific to the information in the chapter or to the age of the children in your family.

After you have reviewed and written goals for all the chapters—including those for children of specific ages in Part II—you can create a combined list of all your goals on page 244.

When you have done that, you are to be congratulated. You have taken the first step in creating a plan for healthy change for your family based on your personal needs, habits, and abilities. Your goals can help you modify your current behaviors and track your success. Specifically, your family can learn to make a few small, permanent changes at a time. Once you are comfortable with them, review and make additional changes—but only after the previous changes are firmly in place.

By taking smaller steps that become new, healthy habits, you can create positive, lasting change. Be patient with yourself on this journey and you'll be amazed at how great your accomplishments can be! The ROAD to success awaits you and your family.

PART I

. . .

*Creating Your Plan
of Action*

Creating Change:
The ROAD to Success

How do you know if you and your family are ready for a lifestyle change? The first step in making lifestyle changes is to develop an awareness of your current health status, eating habits, and activity levels. Keeping food intake records and an exercise diary can help bring about this awareness. The most powerful changes are those that you can make and keep.

It is important to be realistic about the changes you can make and keep. Good nutrition and exercise habits are developed over a lifetime. Staying on the ROAD requires that changes in the food you eat and the way you exercise become part of your daily life. Are there any major life stresses that may make it hard to focus on weight control? If so, set small goals that can help you to improve your health day by day. Take those steps and keep going down the ROAD. A small change that is permanent is better than a big change you can't maintain. Not everyone in your family will be at the same stage at the same time. Often parents are more ready than their children to embark on a weight-loss program. These roadblocks may mean that changing the food in the home may occur gradually. It is important to understand the entire family's attitude toward change in order to avoid the roadblocks along the way.

Next, identify any roadblocks you have. Take time to consider all the outside factors that contribute to your family's ability to commit to a lifelong change. Think honestly about how certain you are that you and your family can stay committed. Ask yourself what kind of stressors may affect your ability to change, the time commitment needed to succeed, and how realistic your goals are.

Finally, set realistic goals and celebrate the successes that you achieve. Each one of these changes can have a powerful impact on the health of your family. This chapter can help you and your family set achievable goals as you get started on the lifelong ROAD to better health.

How ready do you think your family is for change? Use the information you collected on the Family Assessment Tool (you will find a copy of the tool in Appendix A) to answer the following questions and determine how far along the ROAD to success you and your family are.

Where Are You on the ROAD to Successful Change?

YES NO   *Check YES or NO to answer the following questions:*

☐ ☐   Are you willing to limit television and screen time to 2 hours every day?

☐ ☐   Are you willing to be an example and model good eating and exercise behaviors?

☐ ☐   Are you able to commit to working hard every day to change the way the whole family eats, plays, and exercises?

☐ ☐   Has your family discussed food and exercise goals?

☐ ☐   Do you model good eating and exercise behaviors?

☐ ☐   Is your body mass index (BMI) within the normal range?

☐ ☐   Have you started to make changes in the foods you eat?

☐ ☐   Does your family plan weekly menus?

☐ ☐   Have you been successful at weight loss?

☐ ☐   Do you know how to change your eating and exercise habits?

☐ ☐   Have you started an exercise and food plan?

☐ ☐   Does your family eat meals together more than 3 times per week?

_____ *How many yes answers did you have?*

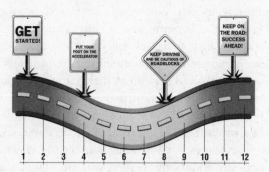

If you answered yes to between 1 and 4 questions, it is time to get your foot on the accelerator and focus on making small changes toward healthier habits. If you scored between 5 and 8, you are on the ROAD to better health, but be careful of those roadblocks. If you scored between 9 and 12, use the tips in this chapter to refine and improve your goals or decisions.

The ROAD to success is a process of change for you and your family. On any road there are roadblocks, detours, and changes in direction. The ROAD requires you and your family to examine some key components essential to making change permanent. What does the ROAD to success involve? Remember, ROAD stands for

- **R**ole modeling
- **O**rganizing and **o**pportunities
- **A**ccess and **a**vailability
- **D**ecisions and goals

Before the journey down the road to success begins, recognize that change can be difficult and your attitude toward change is important. Change is a good news, bad news proposition. The good news for you as a parent is that your child learns to imitate almost everything you do. And the bad news for you as a parent is that your child learns to imitate almost everything you do! This imitation or modeling can be used in a positive way to create a healthy change for your family. This book is about creating a climate of change and changes that you can live with.

A positive attitude, focusing on small changes and gradually improving your health, is the key ingredient for success. It is not about a diet that is short-lived and fails. It is not about giving up all your favorite foods or family activities. It *is* about guiding your family down the ROAD that can affect the family's health for generations to come. If you have a positive attitude about guiding your child with your actions, and you're willing to learn what positive actions to take, the health benefits will follow. In the short run, it is easier to focus on telling your child what to do, but consider over the long term improving your knowledge and habits and showing your child how you do it. In all things, parents are the best teachers. In changing your approach, you will be promoting lifelong and lasting change. Sometimes the change will be easy: sometimes difficult for both you and your family. Your family's attitudes toward the meaning of health and the importance of food and activity all must be examined. Can you focus on the small changes that can make a big difference, or are you looking for a quick fix? Are you ready to begin the journey? Circumstances often limit our ability to make sweeping change, but small changes can be meaningful in the long run. Focus on the small changes that can have a great impact. Go step by step.

Small Changes Are Powerful

Juan is fourteen years old and requires 2,200 calories per day to maintain his weight. As he spends more time with friends, he adds two sodas per day to his intake. Not a problem, right? Wrong! It is a big problem in the long run. He now is consuming 2,500 calories per day, and over a year. This represents approximately a 30-pound weight gain over what would be predicted for his normal growth and development. This process can also work in reverse. Decreasing calories by 100 per day, the equivalent of a medium cookie, can result in a 10-pound weight loss over a year. Small changes do *make a difference.*

Children and adolescents learn by example, and parents are the best role models. Studies show that overweight parents tend to have overweight children. Some of this may be genetic, while some may be the environment the parent creates for the child. Many overweight adults have lower levels of physical activity and unhealthy diets that their children tend to mimic.

It is never too late to change. Change is a gradual process of give and take and negotiating what your family can live with. Throughout this book the activities and planning charts can help guide you in adopting healthier habits for your family. When possible, we make suggestions for ways to work together as a family as you create change.

The ROAD Begins: Role Modeling

Consider your own food choices, family traditions, and beliefs. Chances are much of what you do and consider important you learned through role modeling from your family growing up. Although everyone has heard about role modeling, many parents may not realize how important it is. More and more research is showing links between parents' behaviors about eating and how children react to food and eating.

Take the example of parents feeding their young child peas and saying, "Yummy peas! Eat your peas!" yet never putting any vegetables on their own plates. Picture other parents happily eating their vegetables and showing the child how much they like the taste and also saying, "Yum, I like my broccoli." The impact is even stronger if the parent also shows the positive effects of healthy behaviors, saying. "I feel good after eating my broccoli, and I have lots of energy from eating it. How about we take a bike ride?" Even older children and adolescents learn about choosing healthy foods from their parents. Grabbing an apple as the "original fast food" shows the value of fruits and vegetables better than lecturing about the need to eat them.

That type of modeling shows the child the desired type of behavior (eating vegetables or fruits) and also links it to an appealing benefit of eating vegetables (the energy for a bike ride). This may sound like simple common sense, yet many parents do not realize the importance of modeling this behavior for their children. Instead, they may offer the child dessert if the youngster can manage to "get through" eating the green stuff. This is a way of discouraging eating those vegetables.

You Are the Best Role Model:
Practice What You Preach

Research by Amy Galloway and colleagues indicates that a "tell" rather than "do" philosophy may actually have exactly the opposite effect from the one desired. Pressuring, nagging, or forcing children to eat fruits and vegetables, for example, may cause them to eat less of those foods as well as cause a negative response to the foods. Model the behavior you want, don't lecture. Children remember what you do more than what you say. Work on your own behaviors while trying to change your child and your family.

Many parents are not aware of just how much their children imitate them, from the moment they're born, to when they walk and speak, to when they become parents themselves. The home environment has a huge impact on children, especially when they are young. Parents model not only healthy eating habits but also physical activity throughout childhood and adolescence. In a two-year study, families with low levels of physical activity and a high-calorie diet had daughters with a higher body mass index (BMI), (Appendix B) and body fat levels compared to families with health-promoting behaviors. The Framingham Children's Study revealed that children of active mothers were twice as likely as children of inactive mothers to be active. When both parents were physically active, the children were over five times as likely to be active. Indeed, a recent statement on physical activity from the American Academy of Pediatrics recommends that parents increase their own levels of physical activity in order to become good role models for their children.

> ► ROADBLOCK: Exercise Can Be Fun!
> If physical activity is a challenge for you and your family, discuss ways that you could become more active together. Whether it is biking, walking, or dancing, find ways to incorporate activity into your daily lives. Give gifts that promote activity, such as pogo sticks, hula hoops, and even a pedometer!

In some cases, your children may inspire you to get up and move. If they suggest going out to play, do it! No matter how busy or tired you feel, never pass up the opportunity for physical activity with your child—even a simple walk around the block or tossing a ball can make a strong statement that "together time" is better than staring at a TV. This activity creates a climate where movement and exercise are fun and not a chore.

When it comes to eating, many habits are learned at the age when children first learn to feed themselves, during the first few years of life. At that age, children may observe their parents eating and eat only foods that the parents provide. This is an important time to establish preferences and habits around healthy foods and fitness. As children grow older, food selection and habits continue to be key components of parental role modeling, but other behaviors and concerns are also learned from parents. For example, the older child's body satisfaction is learned in part from the parent's view of his or her own body weight and dieting practices. A study by Beth Abramovitz and Leann Birch indicates that children as young as five are twice as likely to have ideas and concerns about dieting when their mother is dieting. Clearly parents need to model health-promoting behaviors and avoid modeling the latest fad diet or program. A mother's active dieting can also encourage her children to restrain their eating behaviors and ignore internal cues for hunger and fullness. Research by Lori Francis and Leann Birch suggests that a mother's preoccupation with weight and dieting may increase her tendency to restrict her daughters' intake to influence their weight. Boys who are encouraged to diet by their mothers are more likely to attempt unhealthy ways to control weight, such as meal skipping, fasting, or binge eating. The message is clear: Model what you want your child to learn—healthy eating and exercise habits, not dieting! This is an opportunity to reflect on what you are teaching your child about lifelong weight control.

As children grow up, they become more affected by the world beyond their parents, including teachers, peers, and the media. Children who have developed a taste for healthy foods and a firm foundation of healthy habits from good parental role modeling are more likely to remain on that path in the long run.

How Can I Tell If My Child Is Overweight?

Many parents have a hard time determining whether or not their child is overweight. They may have grown up in families where being a "little big" is the norm. Or they may be overly critical, even when their child does not need to slim down.

The Body Mass Index (BMI) provides a more realistic measure of health than weight alone. Calculate BMIs for your whole family using the table in Appendix B.

Parenting Styles

All parents want to provide the best for their children. To this end, keep in mind that supporting and encouraging your child through appropriate role modeling and communication style may be a key strategy to promoting healthy weight. Since children need both structure and support, it is important to develop a balance between nurturance and setting boundaries.

Researchers have identified three basic parenting styles:

- **Authoritative** (nurturing and sets boundaries). These parents explain why rules are important and why children should follow rules. They reason with their children and consider the children's point of view even though they might not agree. They are firm, with kindness, warmth, and caring. They set high standards and encourage their children to be independent. These parents want to promote self-regulation in their children with nurturance.
- **Authoritarian** (little nurturance and sets boundaries). These parents are controlling. They dictate how their children should behave. They stress obedience to authority and discourage discussion. They are demanding and directive. They expect their orders to be obeyed and do not encourage give-and-take. They have low levels of sensitivity and do not expect their children to disagree with their decisions.
- **Permissive** (nurturing with few boundaries set). These parents are accepting and warm but exert little control. They do not set limits, and they allow children to set their own schedules. They do not set expectations for their children.

Review the characteristics in the following two-column list and start to examine what kind of parenting style you use most of the time. The goal of successful parenting is to achieve the right balance between providing boundaries while being nurturing.

NURTURING	SETTING BOUNDARIES
1. I encourage my children to talk about their troubles.	1. I always follow through on discipline for my children, no matter how long it takes.
2. My children and I have warm intimate moments together.	2. I try to make my children behave as they should, most of the time.
3. I encourage my children to be curious, to explore, and to question things.	3. I do not let my children convince me to change my mind after I have refused a request.
4. I find it interesting and educational to be with my children for long periods.	4. Once I decide how to deal with my children's misbehavior, I follow through on it.

(continued)

NURTURING	SETTING BOUNDARIES
5. I make sure my children know that I appreciate what they try to accomplish.	5. I believe that a family rule should be enforced with explanation and discussion.
6. I respect my children's opinions and encourage them to express them.	6. I do not let my children talk me into letting them off more easily than I had intended.

How you communicate with your children and your parenting style may impact their long-term weight. Parents who have a predominantly authoritian style (little nurturance and setting boundaries) have been found to have the highest prevalence of overweight children. In a study of 872 first-grade children, those who had authoritarian mothers had a five times greater risk of becoming overweight than those whose parents were more responsive.

Training Parents to Beat Obesity

Moria Golan, a researcher at the University of Israel, has studied various approaches to helping overweight children. One of her study programs shows that teaching parents to help children develop better eating habits is more effective than teaching children directly. Golan's study found that seven years after ending the program, 60 percent of children in the "parent training" program were nonobese, compared with 31 percent of children in the "child training" program. In essence, Golan's research was targeted toward teaching parents to role-model the behaviors they want in their children.

Parenting Styles and the Role of Parents and Children in Food Selection and Consumption

Authoritative parents can use nurturing and boundary setting to help teach their children how to eat healthily. The parents set the boundaries by deciding what foods are brought into the home and by providing healthy choices for children. They can use meal- and snacktimes to talk about healthy food choices for children. They can also respond to children's cues by allowing them to decide when and how much to eat. In this sense, authoritative parents are teaching their children how to self-regulate food intake, or decide whether to start and when to stop eating.

The ROAD Continues: O Is for Organizing Food Selection

The next step along the ROAD to success is to organize food selections and provide opportunities to improve your health. Good nutrition doesn't just happen; it requires some planning on your part.

Since parents usually purchase the family's groceries, they are in a good position to organize and monitor what foods enter the home. Make sure healthy foods are available in your home by organizing a shopping list prior to going to the store. This means deciding what you will bring home. Stock your home with healthy snacks such as fruits, vegetables, low-fat cheese sticks, low-fat yogurt, whole-grain crackers, and pretzels. Cut up fresh fruit and prepare carrot sticks and low-fat dressing to make sure your children have easy access to such foods. Better yet, place cut-up fresh fruit or vegetable sticks in the refrigerator at your children's eye level, where they can easily see and reach for them.

Older children may be consuming food away from home, so help them review school menus and make the best food choices available that day. Adolescents know what food choices are healthy and rarely need to be advised of the benefits of skim milk versus soda. Suggest to your children that opportunities exist to provide their bodies with nutritious or better choice foods. You may not be able to influence directly what your teen chooses at school, but you are still in charge of the foods brought into the home. Keep in mind that although older children may not appear to be listening, when you give suggestions and explore potential roadblocks, they just might be able to create their own detours!

▶ **ROADBLOCK: How to Set Boundaries Before You Go Shopping**
Parents often struggle with telling their children no when it comes to an endless choice of less healthy foods. Advertisements on television, peers, and the fact that all of us like sweet foods make the task of balancing setting boundaries and nuturing challenging. Head this off at the pass by allowing your children to pick out one less healthy food at the store per week. Give children the opportunity to discuss their favorite foods and participate in organizing the grocery list. Sharing this expectation at home or in the car communicates your family's intent to be healthy without making sweet or fatty foods forbidden.

Avoid keeping an abundance of unhealthy foods in the home. This is easier said than done. Parents struggle with the sugary cereal purchased during a weak moment at the grocery store or grandmother giving bags of candy. If you do face those roadblocks, keep the less healthy foods out of sight and out of reach. For instance, keep cookies on the top shelf of the cabinet. To take an extra step, stock only individually packaged cookies or other snack-type foods so that portion control is easier when these foods are allowed as part of a balanced eating plan.

Navigating the Grocery Store

If parents choose healthy foods for their family, such as fresh fruits and vegetables, whole grains, lean meats, and low-fat dairy products, then junk food and soda simply are not available at home.

Shopping together can be a great opportunity for parents to teach their children how to navigate the grocery store, or it can be a battle of wills. Most families bring their children to the store with them after work or on weekends when it is more convenient. Prepare yourself and your children to resist temptation by making sure no one is hungry when you set foot in the store. Allow your young children to have their own "fruit and vegetable" cart, especially reserved for fresh produce. Most of the foods that provide the most nutrition are found on the outside aisles of the store. So organize your shopping adventure to hit the produce section first and fill up their basket. Older children may be less interested in going to the store with you, but have them organize their list of favorite fruits, vegetables, and healthy snacks before you leave for shopping. These strategies communicate that you value your children's opinion after you have established the ground rules. Young children are not capable of making all good choices on their own; they need your guidance to set boundaries in making good choices.

Getting your children involved in making smart choices can be turned into a fun game. Instead of saying, "You can't have that chocolate cookie," allow your children to choose between two healthier options for snacks, such as graham crackers or animal crackers. However, remember that as the parent, you are in charge and you definitely can say no to your child's unhealthy choices. Stand your ground and set rules about what food items are allowed. (See Appendix B: Healthy Shopping List for a list that's easy to follow.)

Parents usually prepare most of the food for the family too. This makes them responsible for selecting healthy cooking methods, such as grilling, steaming, baking, or sautéing instead of frying. If your children are old enough to help with food preparation, try to involve them in learning these healthy cooking methods. Working families often struggle with the concept of a healthy meal after a long day at work, with homework lurking around the corner. Remember, a healthy meal can be as simple as a sandwich, fruit salad, and pretzels. If your budget allows, purchase cut-up fruit or bag salads. Keep canned fruit in its own juice and frozen vegetables on hand for quick meal preparation. (For more ideas on how to make your meals healthier, see Appendix B: Low-Fat Recipe Substitutions.)

Timmy is an eleven-year-old boy. His parents have noticed that his clothes are starting to fit a little snugly. They take him to the doctor, who tells them that his BMI is above the 95th percentile for his age. That night, Timmy's parents do some research on problems caused by being overweight, and what they find scares them. They don't want their child to be unhealthy in the future. They become aware that they bear the responsibility for what food is brought into the home and that change is needed in the family's grocery list. Timmy and his parents organize a list of things they know they can change. These simple changes include the following:

USUAL	NEW
Whole milk	*2% milk*
Chips	*Pretzels*
Ranch salad dressing	*Reduced-fat dressing*
Ice cream	*Sugar-free Popsicles*

Although the changes are not huge, the calorie savings for Timmy are significant, since he consumes those foods every day. They allow him to save 600 calories each day without dieting or having his parents control his intake. These simple changes provide the opportunity for the family to improve Timmy's health.

The A Along the ROAD:
Access and Availability

Scheduling consistent meal- and snacktimes, especially for younger children, is important. When children are allowed free access to the refrigerator and pantry, they are more likely to snack before and after dinner, which can lead to excess calorie intake. By eliminating "grazing" throughout the day, children are better able to identify when they are hungry and when they are full.

Parents can help their children make healthy choices and can avoid being too controlling by making certain that healthy choices are available and accessible. According to research done by Tom Baranowski at the USDA Children's Nutrition Research Center, "availability and accessibility" are the key components in increasing the fruits and vegetables children consume. Because parents are the gatekeepers in the home, they can control which foods are brought into the home. But if healthy foods are in the cupboard out of sight, or are too difficult for children to prepare, children probably won't eat them. This is the difference between availability and accessibility. The foods may be in the home and thus available but not easy enough to get, or accessible.

For example, having apples already sliced and placed on a plate where the child can easily grab them makes them more accessible. Or cut celery into sticks and put them on a plate with peanut butter, so your child eats them instead of potato chips.

At the same time that you provide more of these healthy options, you should decrease the availability of unwanted foods, such as soda, chips, and cookies. Picture the typical adolescent coming home after school. If she opens the fridge and the first thing she sees is fruit that's already washed and ready to eat and chilled bottles of water, she's more likely to go ahead and have that—especially if no soda and chips are in the cupboard (or if the soda is warm and the chips are up on a high shelf).

> ▶ ROADBLOCK: Grazing
> *Grazing* refers to the habit of wandering around freely with food, so that eating occurs throughout the day, often without awareness of how much one is eating. Grazing also represents a permissive form of parenting: allowing your children to roam with food wherever they chose.

A healthy approach is to provide smaller, more frequent feedings throughout the day, such as three meals and one or two small snacks, with limits to how many snacks. This strategy provides structured access to healthy foods. Establishing such eating behaviors at an early age helps children naturally follow the eating patterns as they grow older. Parents and caretakers must also establish where meals and snacks are to be eaten. For example, children should eat meals and snacks at the table and not in front of the television. The family also should sit at the table and eat together at mealtimes, without turning on the TV. Older children, who may eat as much as half their food away from home, present a new set of challenges. The provision of breakfast—and making time for this in the hectic morning schedule—is crucial to long-term success. In fact, people who consume breakfast, and particularly a low-sugar cereal, have better nutrient intakes and lower BMIs. A low-sugar whole-grain cereal gives your children access to the healthy food, and placing the box of cereal on the table the night before makes it available quickly on busy mornings.

Remember, parents provide the healthy meals and snacks and set the boundaries for what is being brought into the home. Let your children choose what and how much they want to eat from the nutritious foods served. However, if your children decide to skip the vegetables served and request second helpings of starches, like mashed potatoes and pasta, or ask for dessert instead, you must establish and enforce the rules you have set. For example, make a family rule that before seconds or dessert is served, both children and parents must eat at least one bite of all the foods on their dinner plate. This helps to ensure that your family is eating balanced meals and to prevent overeating of less healthy foods.

▶ HELPFUL HINT: **Make the Choice Easier for Your Child: A Recipe for Success**
Cook enough for one portion each of your child's favorite starches, such as macaroni and cheese. Preplate the foods in the kitchen and refrigerate the leftovers. Model this behavior for your children. You can even use it as a game to help them learn math!

The ROAD Continues: D Is for Decisions and Goals

The decisions that need to be made along the ROAD to success include how you are going to communicate with your family about weight, healthy eating, and exercise. When roadblocks are discovered, what decisions will your family make and what goals will you set to improve the health of your family for years to come?

How to communicate with your children about health, nutrition, and weight depends on how old they are and their health status. Our society values thinness, and our children are exposed to media images and visions of what is ideal. At the same time, two-thirds of Americans are overweight. We are exposed to large volumes of great-tasting food and then told not to eat it. These challenges are substantial.

Home should be a haven where children have their needs met. These needs include love and acceptance regardless of their weight. All members of the family should respect certain guidelines so that needed behavior change can occur in a safe environment. If your children are overweight, chances are they have been teased or made fun of at school or by friends. They need to feel safe at home. If your child says, "Susie said I am fat," listen, don't lecture or dismiss the claim. Ask questions that require more than a yes or no answer. These include "Why do you think Susie said that?" or "What do you think about that?" Your questions should open the door for solutions rather than ridicule or dismiss what the child is feeling.

As young children are learning to eat, they are also learning whether or not to pay attention to their body's cues about when to start and stop eating. Young children are attuned naturally to their nutritional needs. They typically regulate their energy intake well, without their parents' control. Demanding that your children clean their plates assumes that you know how much food it takes to fill your children up. Avoid the temptation to overfeed by serving your children on smaller plates and allowing them to ask for more if they are still hungry. Your best communication strategy is to model healthy eating. Serve yourself moderate portions and choose a variety of foods.

As Your Children Grow and Develop, Set Up a Reward System for Good Behavior That Is Independent of Food

Avoid using food as a reward or punishment. We all need food to fuel our bodies, and viewing food as a reward or punishment may not help us choose the best fuel wisely. Instead, have a nonfood system for reaching goals. Motivate your children by using rewards such as stickers, small toys, or a trip to the park. If negative behaviors require punishment, use restrictions like taking away privileges, such as telephone or TV time. Older children and adolescents require a different system of rewards for good behavior. These may be tangible, like a gift card to the movies, or simply recognition of hard work. Sincere praise and acknowledgment for a job well done is a simple form of positive reinforcement.

Help your children learn to have a healthy balance. Being too restrictive about eating fatty foods or sugary snacks may lead to unwanted results. Parents who limit junk food to the extreme may lead their children to overeat when they have the opportunity, harming their ability to self-regulate.

Instead, limit the availability of less healthy foods without cutting them off completely. One way to do this is to limit them to designated days or times. For example, agree to have dessert only one night a week, or to have soda with dinner on Saturday evenings instead of every night.

Serve Healthy Foods in Positive Contexts

Take a moment to think about how people usually serve sweets. Birthday parties always feature cake as the grand finale, and special occasions almost always include some type of dessert. People learn to associate sugar and fat with good times.

Start to focus on serving healthy foods, such as fruit and veggies, in positive contexts. For example, include several of your child's favorite fruits and vegetables at their special event or party. Or, instead of serving sweets for dessert every night, switch to serving fruit. It helps to have several varieties to choose from, so that children can pick their favorite and "own" it. Enabling children to feel in control about which fruits or veggies they eat creates a more positive attitude about those foods.

Terms like *good, bad,* or *junk* often come from the media trying to get you to buy food from one company and not another. But labeling foods causes a preoccupation with eating and food. Try using terms such as *less healthy* or *those foods that we eat occasionally.* Acknowledge that these foods taste good rather than applying a label of *junk food.*

Most people who feel they can't have something, soon start craving more of it. And being too extreme about *good food* can turn your child away from healthy food. Total, overall food intake is what's important— not just one food or meal that you or your children consume. If you worry about every single item your children eat—especially if you comment on it—you run the risk of having your children tune out everything you say, or sneaking food when you aren't around. Remember to evaluate your parenting style. Do what you believe is best for your family when making healthy choices, but don't berate your children for occasionally enjoying a favorite treat.

Setting Goals for You and Your Family

The first step in making a plan is to set goals. The goals are going to tell you *what* you are aiming for. The plan is going to tell you *how* you are going to meet those goals you set for yourself. Goals can be both long-term and short-term. Short-term goals are the little steps that help you get to the long-term goal. You can think of it like a set of monkey bars. The long-term goal is to reach the other side without falling; the short-term goal is to reach each little bar along the way. Long-term goals can be three months from now, a year from now, or ten years from now.

When it comes to slimming down, your child may not actually need to lose weight. Depending on your child's age and size, he or she may benefit from simply cutting back on calories and exercising more. A realistic short-term goal for your child may be to maintain his or her current weight while continuing to grow. A doctor or a registered dietitian can help develop your child's specific goal. However, depending on your child's weight, your primary care physician may deem a weight loss of ½ to 2 pounds a week medically necessary. Make sure you get the advice of a doctor and a registered dietitian if you and your child's goal is for the child to lose weight. The plan for losing weight should include both exercise and nutritional changes, as it is the balance of food and exercise that determine weight gain or loss.

Whatever your child's goal, the entire family must be supportive. Singling out an overweight child at mealtime can be embarrassing and can make it harder to build your child's confidence about making healthful eating choices and changes in lifestyle. Remember, making healthy eating choices is beneficial for *everyone*. Other children in your home will also learn and carry these habits into adulthood.

Creating a reward system is the last part of the plan. A reward system can be helpful in motivating children and family to stick to the plan and accomplish those goals that you set. It helps to know what your children value most in order to set a reward.

> ▶ HELPFUL HINT: **Professionals Can Help**
> If you have tried to create change but find it difficult to do so and would like extra support, seek some help. Registered dietitians are the food and nutrition experts. To find a registered dietitian in your area, visit www.eatright.org, the Web site for the American Dietetic Association.

Be sure to include your children in the project of coming up with goals, setting up a plan, and developing the reward system. If children help to develop these, they will be much more willing to participate. If you set up the goals, plans, and rewards without them, you may find it almost impossible to motivate them to follow through.

Sample Goals

Long-term goal:	I will lose 12 pounds in 3 months.
Short-term goals:	I will decrease my soda intake to one per week. I will increase walking time by 15 minutes a day.
Parent long-term goal:	I will provide healthier food options for my family by adding five new recipes per month.
Parent short-term goals:	I will reduce the number of fast-food meals to one per week. I will purchase only sugar-free drinks for our family to drink at home.

Guidelines for Goal Setting

When planning what you want to achieve, follow these simple guidelines:

- Make your goals realistic.
- Modify your goals if you find that they are unrealistic.
- Set more than one goal. These may include a food goal and an exercise goal. (Use the Family Goals in Appendix A to help set your goals.)
- Give yourself specific goals with specific time frames. For example, to set a fitness goal, first find a starting point or baseline for your activity and endurance level. If the activity you choose is walking, determine how far and for how long you can walk the first time you perform the activity. You might start by timing yourself when walking once around the block. Say that takes you 15 minutes. Then you can set your goal based on this information. Your goal might be to walk faster, eventually to go twice around the block in 20 minutes. Or you might aim to walk for 30 minutes without stopping.
- Make your goals functional and meaningful.
- Make the goals appropriate for the age or ability of each family member.

  - A goal for a three-year-old might be increasing the amount of playtime that the child participates in each day (this does not include watching TV or playing video games). The goal might be a developmental goal, such as being able to ride a push toy to the end of the block and back home.
  - A goal for a six-year-old might be to learn to ride a bike without training wheels.
  - A goal for a ten-year-old might be to ride a bike for 20 minutes.
  - A goal for a teenager might be to walk or run for 20 minutes.
- Plan a reward for when the goal is accomplished.

Establishing Rewards

If you have more than one child, your reward for each one may be different. For example, Timmy likes money, but Bobby likes to spend extra time at the park. If the reward you set is not something they are interested in, they will not be motivated to accomplish the goal.

Since you are trying to associate success and feeling good with things other than eating, remember to explore nonfood rewards. Rewards can be anything from verbal praise to a toy.

Simple Rewards

- verbal praise
- hugs
- kisses
- stickers
- money (in small amounts)
- toys
- activities, such as bowling or biking
- playing at the park
- going to a movie
- iTunes gift card
- movie gift card

Your children, as well as your family, will find it is fun to keep track of when each short-term goal is achieved. Keeping track is very important to helping you and your children recognize and feel good about the success, even a small one.

▶ **HELPFUL HINT: Charting Success**
Tracking with a chart that is posted somewhere in the house has been found to be useful by many families. The Family Goals in Appendix A provide a form you can use to chart your goals and view your successes.

Sample Goals and Plan

Long-Term Goal: Exercise
By the end of the month:

- I will ride my bike to my friend's house and back, three times a week (about 20 minutes).
- I will walk with Mom, Dad, and Snoopy around the park three times a week (about 30 minutes).
- I will limit the amount of time spent in front of the computer or television to 1 hour per day.

Long-Term Goal: Nutrition
By the end of the month:

- I will recognize portions sizes that are appropriate for my age.
- I will not eat fast foods more than 1 time per week (4 times a month).
- I will replace all of my regular soda with diet soda.
- I will eat fruit for dessert at dinner instead of sweets.

Rewards
- For each short-term goal achieved, I will receive a free pass for extra time at the park.
- When I achieve two short-term goals, I will receive $2.
- When I achieve a long-term goal and maintain it for 3 weeks, I can purchase a toy under $10.

Identifying Benefits and Roadblocks

The next activity is to make a benefits and barriers list. As with a pros and cons list, draw a line vertically down the middle of the page and label one side *Benefits* and the other *Roadblocks*. In the *Benefits* column, help your family list the good things about exercising and losing weight. In the *Roadblocks* column, help your family think of things that could prevent them from exercising and losing weight. This activity will help bring up any problems they feel they have and point out areas that need to be worked out (such as transportation to sports practice). Knowing what the challenges are can help you solve the problems or at least become aware of them as they occur.

What Could Happen If We Try to Change?

BENEFITS	ROADBLOCKS
• I will be able to run faster on the soccer field.	• Soccer practice is Tuesdays, but Mom works late that night—no ride.
• I will be able to fit into my clothes that are now too small.	• I get short of breath when I exercise/play.
• Kids may stop teasing me.	• My friends eat lots of junk food when I am around. I usually have some too.
• I will have better overall health.	
• If we measure food portions, we will save money and not waste food.	

Believe You Can Do It!

"I think I can, I think I can, I think I can" is a lesson everyone recalls learning from the *Little Engine That Could*. That story teaches that you can accomplish anything you put your mind to. The little blue engine stopped to help the train that was carrying a bunch of toys for the kids on the other side of the mountain.

Everyone thought that because the blue engine was so little he wouldn't be able to carry the heavy load, but he told himself that he could do it, and he did it!

Believing in yourself is a crucial piece of the "change" puzzle, especially when it comes to improving any kind of health behavior, whether it is to quit smoking, floss daily, exercise, or eat healthier.

Self-Confidence: It's About Believing

The little engine in the story had high self-confidence because he believed he could make it up the mountain. What do you think would have happened if the train believed all the others and told himself he couldn't make it up the mountain?

Recent studies show that having high self-confidence actually affects the outcome of your task. For example, people who believed they could quit smoking were more likely actually to quit and maintain the healthier behavior than those who didn't. Restricting calories, making healthier food choices, and increasing physical activities are all areas in which you can achieve when you believe.

Alesha and her family have recently developed a family health plan. Part of the plan includes being physically active every day after school for at least 30 minutes, but Alesha doesn't believe she can really do that because she feels so tired when she gets home from school. Alesha tells her sister, "I don't think I can do it for even a week."

Alesha's sister encourages her by offering to walk around the block with her every day after school. After two weeks, Alesha realizes that she feels much better after walking, and that the tired feeling she has after school is no longer there! She notices she can even concentrate on her homework better. Alesha now thinks, "I can do this and it's easy!" To this day, she continues to walk around the block every day after school.

With trial and error, you will find what works best for motivating your child and yourself. Be sure to follow these same methods for yourself. Create your own goals, plans, and list of rewards. Share them with your child. You will serve as a positive role model and offer your child an opportunity to lend you support too.

Make your planning and your success a team effort!

Setting Your Family's Goals

The table that follows is a sample to show you how to keep track of your goals in the various categories that can help improve your family's health and weight. As you create goals for each of the chapters, enter them on the "master" table in Appendix A. This is the basis of your plan for creating change.

Down the left-hand side are categories focusing on changing habits, food choices, and fitness levels. Use the remaining spaces to enter information about individual children; the age-based chapters will help you focus on actions that will help your children. Remember to add your goals for improving communication too!

FAMILY GOALS

	Family	Adults	Child 1	Child 2
Parenting Goal Specific goal: Measure: Time frame:	I will have two healthy snacks for my children to choose from every day after school	I will role-model healthy eating by eating a veg-etable every night at dinner		
Healthy Behaviors Goal Specific goal: Measure: Time frame:				
Healthy Food Goal Specific goal: Measure: Time frame:				
Fitness Goal Specific goal: Measure: Time frame:				

Go to Appendix A for a full-size copy.

Fiction: Being overweight doesn't have anything to do with overeating. I don't eat nearly as much as other people, but I still gain weight.

Fact: You can't judge what you need by looking at someone else—your body has its own unique needs. Different individuals eat different amounts because their metabolic rates are different, but the basic reason for obesity is overeating. Biology differs between individuals and their needs, but in all cases, eating too much leads to being overweight.

2

• • •

Smart Behaviors to Start
Slimming Down

Let's get started! Losing weight and getting fit is a process, and small changes do make a big difference. Throughout this chapter, you will find suggestions for ways to lose weight and get fit. Depending on you and your family's needs, you may find that some are easy for you and others aren't suited to your particular situation. Let's throw the old notion out that you must be miserable to lose weight. Small changes that you can live with over time can have a big impact.

One thing is certain: Seeing progress makes it easier to continue making positive changes. This chapter offers simple steps for getting started on the right track to a healthier life. To assess how far along the ROAD to success you and your family are, answer the following questions.

Where Are You on the ROAD to Healthy Behaviors?

YES NO   *Check YES or NO to answer the following questions:*

☐ ☐ Do you plan meal- and snacktimes for you and your family?

☐ ☐ Do you eat three meals a day and avoid skipping meals?

☐ ☐ Do you pack a lunch for school or work?

☐ ☐ Do you read food labels?

☐ ☐ Do you allow your children to choose how much to eat?

☐ ☐ Do you role-model healthy eating habits?

☐ ☐ Do you reward healthy behaviors with nonfood items?

☐ ☐ Do you eat without the TV on?

☐ ☐ Do you have healthy snacks available and accessible?

☐ ☐ Do you preportion food so that you don't have to be restrictive with your children or yourself?

☐ ☐ Do you role-model staying active?

☐ ☐ Do you exercise as a family?

_____ *How many yes answers did you have?*

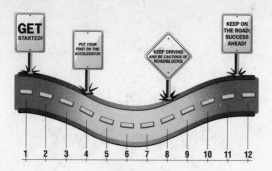

If you scored between 1 and 4, it is time to get your foot on the accelerator and focus on small changes toward healthier habits. If you scored between 5 and 8, you are on the ROAD to better habits, but watch out for those roadblocks. If you scored between 9 and 12, use the tips in this chapter to refine and improve your goals or decisions.

Healthy Habits

There's more to changing your weight and fitness than going on a diet. The experts agree that for weight management to be successful, you must commit to lifelong healthy behaviors that include good eating and ongoing physical activity.

Having the healthy body you want—and keeping it—means making changes in your behavior. Developing healthy eating habits during young childhood and adolescence will not only help prevent chronic health problems such as diabetes, obesity, high blood pressure, and heart disease but also will set the pace for a lifetime of healthy behaviors. Following are some simple actions for establishing healthy habits. As simple as these are, be patient with yourself—change isn't always easy and it doesn't happen overnight. Remember, small changes, like whether you decide not to skip meals or to start an exercise program, can have a big impact over time by making change a habit.

Plan Ahead for Meals and Snacks
as Much as Possible

Children do better with structure and routine. Most children need to eat every two to four hours, so three meals plus two healthy snacks a day are plenty.

Plan ahead so that your children do not graze on unhealthy snacks throughout the day. For example, if you know you are going to be out and about during lunchtime, pack a sandwich and a piece of fruit so you or your child can avoid buying candy bars and chips from a vending machine or fast-food mart.

Don't Skip Meals

It is a myth that skipping meals will help you lose weight. Research associates meal skipping with obesity. The fact is that skipping meals is likely to cause you to overeat at the next meal or to make poor choices in between meals. Allowing yourself or your children to get too hungry makes choosing healthy foods difficult. Think of a time when you were really hungry. What did you choose, an apple or a candy bar? Most people would choose a candy bar, as this type of food makes you feel better in the short run, but the calories would be better spent if you chose an apple, which would also hold you over until mealtime better. Saving 100 to 150 calories would be an added bonus! Try to eat meals and snacks at the same time each day. By eating regularly each day, you have more control over how much you eat by eating only when it is time to eat.

Breakfast: Getting Your Day Started Without Roadblocks

The first roadblock of the day is skipping breakfast. Many people skip breakfast, saying they don't have time to eat or they are not hungry—without having any idea how important it is. Although you may not feel hungry in the morning, it doesn't mean your body does not need the fuel. In fact, children, due to their higher metabolic rate, often have a poor appetite in the morning.

Many nutrition experts believe that breakfast may be the most crucial meal of the day because it provides your body with energy and other necessary nutrients to get the day started and keep it going. By avoiding fasting, you can prevent overeating at lunch or snacking on high-calorie and high-fat snacks late in the morning.

According to the American Dietetic Association, studies show that children who eat breakfast tend to have better total nutrient intake compared with those who skip breakfast. According to a study by Anna Maria Siega-Riz and colleagues, the total calories consumed at breakfast have remained about the same over time in the United States, and the quality of foods consumed at breakfast has improved. Unfortunately, breakfast consumption itself has decreased, especially among adolescents. Given that skipping breakfast has been associated with obesity in the Bogalusa Heart Study, it is wise to encourage breakfast. Children also do better in school when they eat breakfast. The American Dietetic Association suggests that children who eat breakfast are more likely to

- meet daily nutritional needs
- keep their weight under control
- have lower blood cholesterol levels

- attend school more frequently
- make fewer trips to the school nurse's office complaining of tummy aches

Mornings for families are hectic and chaotic. Waking children from deep sleep and getting them out of bed is challenging enough. Next you have children trying to find socks and shoes, pets that need to be fed, and lunches to be made. Adding breakfast to the chaos seems next to impossible. But it can be done! Try these tips to make sure breakfast is a part of your family's day:

- Wake up earlier to prepare and eat breakfast.
- Prepare breakfast the night before (e.g., cut fruit, get the table set, put the cereal on the table).
- Pack an extra half sandwich, piece of fruit, cereal bar, yogurt, or string cheese in your children's lunch for them to eat on the way to school.
- Keep plenty of ready-to-go foods—such as granola bars, cereal bars, trail mix, peanut butter crackers, and milk boxes—in the pantry for those mornings when you really are short on time.

▶ HELPFUL HINT: Cereal—A Simple Solution

Too busy for a big breakfast? Fortified breakfast cereal is an excellent way to start the day. Not only does it provide many nutrients the body needs, cereal is an easy and satisfying food for most children and adults. Choose skim or low-fat (1%) milk to make cereal an even healthier, less fatty choice. You can even eat it dry on the run!

Take Your Lunch with You

Many children participate in the National School Breakfast and Lunch Programs. Often, these meals are not just less expensive but also much healthier than the snack foods in the school's à la carte line or vending machines.

School cafeterias try hard to offer low-fat choices. Suggest that your child look for the healthier choices on the school breakfast and lunch menus, such as these typical alternatives:

- cereal and low-fat milk
- turkey or tuna sandwich
- grilled chicken sandwich
- fresh fruit or fruit cup

- salad with low-calorie dressing
- vegetables without added fat

When given a choice in the lunch line, however, most kids tend to choose the higher-fat items. To help your children avoid that temptation, start sending lunch from home. If this doesn't fit your children's school culture, help them to make the best choices at school or make adjustments in your evening meal planning.

Ask your children to suggest what to include in the packed lunch, but guide them toward more nutritious choices. You also can control portion sizes and limit the number of fattening or sugary snacks. If you're not used to the routine of packing a lunch, start out by trying it a few times a week.

As a parent you can set an example by packing your own healthy lunch to take to work. Being consistent with your behaviors while encouraging healthy food choices for your children will help them form healthier eating habits.

Smart Choices Cut Down Calories in School Lunches

HIGHER-CALORIE/FAT SCHOOL LUNCH	LOWER-CALORIE/FAT SCHOOL LUNCH
Cheeseburger	Grilled chicken sandwich
French fries with ketchup	Salad with low-calorie dressing
Chocolate chip cookie	Fruit cup
Whole milk	Skim milk
Calories: 825	Calories: 535
Fat: 47 g	Fat: 13 g

Share a Daily Meal

Ask yourself how many meals your family ate together last week. When you didn't eat together, what types of foods did you choose? According to a study led by M. W. Gillman, children who regularly eat family meals eat an average of almost one more serving of fruits and vegetables, as well as other helpful nutrients, including fiber, folate, calcium, iron, and vitamins B_6, B_{12}, C, and E. They also eat smaller amounts of saturated and trans fat, soda, and fried foods. One theory is that home-cooked meals are prepared in healthier ways and provide a more balanced mix of nutritious foods. The family meal is more important than just the food choices.

Eat Proper Portion Sizes

Portion sizes of foods have increased substantially over the years. With the arrival of "super-size" and "value-size" meals, most Americans have grown accustomed to larger portions. If you order the super-size to save money, consider splitting it between two family members. But "value" in terms of saving money does not mean it has a high health value.

Studies by Leann Birch and Barbara Rolls showed that when children are served a larger portion, they tend to eat more.

▶ **HELPFUL HINT: Don't Serve It "Family Style"**
When eating at home, you can avoid serving large portions by filling plates in the kitchen and then carrying them to the table, instead of serving foods family style in big bowls at the dinner table, making seconds an easy temptation.

Use a Smaller Plate

Overlarge portions are one of the biggest causes of overeating. Using a smaller plate (e.g., the salad plate instead of the dinner plate) encourages portion control—psychologically you will feel as if you are eating a big meal if you have a full plate of food. To control intake of higher-calorie foods at mealtime, try using the "plate method" shown below.

USE YOUR PLATE TO EAT RIGHT!

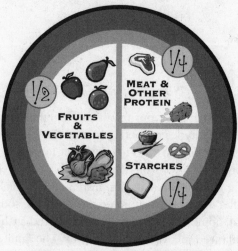

Created by: Pamela Sheridan. Dietetic Intern, © 2007.

The **"plate method"** is simple:

- ½ plate of veggies/fruit
- ¼ plate of lean meat
- ¼ plate of a starch (pasta, rice, bread) or starchy vegetable (potato, corn, peas)

Eat Slowly and at the Table

Eating at the table is a healthy eating habit that you should encourage as soon as table foods are introduced. By eating at the table, you make time to eat. Put your fork down between bites to slow down your eating. While teaching your children good table behaviors, have them practice putting their fork down too—help make it a lifelong habit. Chew each bite of food at least ten times to help slow down eating time. Eating in a hurry leads to overeating, which leads to overweight.

It takes approximately 20 minutes for your brain to receive a message from your stomach that you are full. By taking time to sit down and relax, you stay attuned to satiety cues (the signal from the brain to the stomach that the stomach is full) and prevent overeating. If you are still hungry after 20 minutes, serve yourself seconds of the lower-calorie food—veggies.

Don't Eat with the TV On

It's easy to overeat when you are paying attention to the TV instead of your body and your food. Increased television viewing while eating has been associated with increased calorie intake and being or becoming overweight. Family mealtime is a great opportunity to interact and communicate and for parents to be role models for their children. So turn off the television, pay attention to your satiety cues, and enjoy your family at mealtime.

▶ ROADBLOCK: Timing Your Communication

Mealtime is not the time to remind your children of their shortcomings. Don't lecture about portion sizes, schoolwork, or chores. This is a time to enjoy each other's company, making mealtime a positive experience. If you want your child to enjoy mealtime, keep the doors of communication wide open.

Keep Food Out of Sight

The eye can definitely become bigger than the stomach when foods are left out and visible. Just seeing food makes many people feel hungry or think they feel hungry. If you do keep food out, make it fresh fruit to encourage healthy snacking if your children actually are hungry.

Don't Overly Restrict Food

Overly restricting foods can cause children to sneak foods or to overeat when they are offered treats. Also, children may feel punished or rejected when foods are overly restricted. Food should not have this kind of meaning. Eating should be pleasurable. The best approach is to encourage moderation in eating all types of foods.

▶ ROADBLOCK: How to Promote Healthier Food Choices
When Not Everyone in the Family Is on Board
Is this your family? Fred is a hardworking dad who believes he is entitled to his favorite chips when he comes home from work despite the fact that his daughter Connie is struggling with her weight. He wants the food in the house, but you know it's hard for her not to eat chips when Dad is. To avoid family conflict, a compromise might be one of the following:

- Keep the chips on the highest shelf, out of sight and out of mind for the kids.
- Agree not to eat them in front of the children.
- Eat them on the way home from work.
- Package the snacks in individual bags to control calories.

Avoid Emotional or Boredom Eating

Target your trouble times for eating by keeping a journal of your daily activities and eating habits, and do the same for your children. How many times have you come home feeling exhausted, thinking that if only you had a snack you would feel refreshed and refueled, so you reach for a soda and chips?

If you find that you tend to eat high-calorie snacks when you first get home from work, make sure to have healthier options, like carrots and celery sliced and ready to eat, in the fridge. If you find that your children tend to indulge in snacks after school, have healthy foods available for them as well. One other way to prevent overindulging is to schedule an activity during that time.

Encourage active playtime, such as playing catch in the backyard, instead of computer games or sedentary activities—when eating is all too easy. You could set aside this part of the day as "choretime," when you work together to get some tasks out of the way before dinner—or use the time to make a healthy dinner together.

Keeping a journal not only shows trouble spots; it also helps you track the progress you and your children make.

Parents as Action Heroes

Increase Activity; Decrease "Downtime"

The human body was not designed to be inactive. It was designed for movements like bending, walking, running, skipping, and jumping. Hippocrates, the father of medicine, said, "That which is used, develops; that which is not used, wastes away." That's one reason why keeping the body moving is more beneficial than staying sedentary.

Inactivity leads to muscle *atrophy*, which means the muscles get smaller and weaker. Muscles burn calories the best, so the more muscles you have and the stronger they are, the easier it is to maintain a steady body weight. Children who are sedentary use only the muscles required for lying down, sitting, and walking, and not many muscles are required for that!

Working all the major muscle groups, which occurs when you are physically active, also helps develop your lungs, heart, and body cells. That's another reason why it's important to engage in a variety of activities; to challenge different muscle groups and organs with different activities.

The body becomes stagnant when not in motion. Have you noticed how stiff and sluggish you feel after riding in a car for several hours? That's because your body is designed to be in motion. In other words, when you have to sit for long periods—fidget! Move your feet, stretch your arms, wiggle your legs, and shift positions.

Sedentary activities over long periods of time—like watching television, talking on the phone, and playing computer games—cut into physical activity time. Numerous studies have also shown that people tend to snack more when doing sedentary activities. So not only is the inactivity making the body sluggish (decreasing the energy level), the snacking is increasing calorie intake, which leads to weight gain.

Additional studies have shown that television viewing influences snacking choices. TV watchers see cookies, cakes, chips, and candy bars dance across their screen, and most of these snack choices are high in fat or sugar.

Avoid sitting down for too long, especially in front of the TV. The American Academy of Pediatrics recommends that children over the age of two years old watch no more than two hours of TV a day. For younger children, TV time is not recommended.

Build Physical Activity into Your Daily Routine

Not everyone is interested in sports or intense exercise, but that shouldn't prevent you from engaging in physical activity. (Learn more about the difference between physical activity and exercise in Chapter 4.)

Increasing your physical activity level doesn't mean that you need to become an athlete. In fact, you can activate your day by asking yourself: "If I am sitting, can I add some movement to what I am doing?" For example, most people tend to sit or lie down while talking on the phone. Instead, use the time while you're talking on the phone to stand up. If you are standing while you talk on the phone, you can pace around. Sitting burns approximately 30 to 50 calories an hour (depending on your height, weight, age, and muscle mass), while standing burns approximately 60 to 110 calories an hour, and a slow walk burns approximately 120 to 200 calories an hour. If you can increase your calories burned by just 250 calories a day, seven days a week, you burn a total of 1,750 calories a week—about half a pound of weight loss. That equals approximately 26 lost pounds in one year!

Movement of any type is better than nonmovement like lying and sitting. Make an assessment of your day (at the bottom of the Daily Food Record in Appendix A). How often during the day are you sitting? How can you add some movement to that sitting time?

Get Physically Active as a Family

The family is at the core of a child's world, thinking, and habits. Children learn from their parents, making it crucial for parents to set a good example.

Enjoying physical activity together as a family can create a surprising amount of quality time for parents and children. The activity does not have to be sports related, if that's not your style. You can play tag, chase the dog, play Twister or hula hoop or jump rope. You can make up your own games with your own rules. Get creative and have fun with it!

Also, activity doesn't need to take a huge chunk of time. Start with 15- to 20-minute sessions three times a week. What you choose to do is not as important as getting up and moving (instead of being sedentary) together. You'll be amazed at how much fun you can have as a family—and you'll see your energy level increase. Mark time on the family calendar to have fun and play together.

For parents with teens, be sensitive to your teens' needs. Typically, adolescents and teens tend to separate from their families, so don't take it too personally if your teens don't want to participate in family time. The main goal is to get teens moving—whether they're alone or with friends.

▶ ROADBLOCK: No Time, Not Safe, Too Hot

Wondering what you are going to do when it is raining? What if it is not safe for your children to be outside when you are not around? A few ideas you can suggest include hula-hooping or jumping rope on a porch or open space indoors. How about dancing to your favorite music or running in place while you watch your favorite television show after school? Get your children moving by using a low stool or a step to do step aerobics. Make sure that your children stay active and can get exercise from an assortment of activities.

▶ HELPFUL HINT: Laugh Away the Fat

Did you know that smiling and laughing produce chemicals in the body that help increase your energy level? A study conducted by Maciej Buchowski and colleagues concluded that genuine laughter can increase energy expenditure by 10 to 20 percent. For example, 10 to 15 minutes of laughter a day could burn up to 40 calories. That doesn't sound like much, but in one year's time that would be the equivalent of 4 pounds lost just by laughing.

So enjoying activity can help you feel better and also burn a few extra calories while you're at it.

Make Change a Habit

Small changes can have a big impact. Habits take time to make, and it takes time to unmake bad habits. Changing habits also takes practice, lots of it. Changing a habit is much like learning to ride a bike or hit a tennis ball. There will be many failures before you learn the skill and become proficient. Actions need to be repeated over and over again before they become comfortable and can start becoming a new habit. Small, consistent changes over time are easier to handle than large, difficult changes. Focus on one small goal at a time. For example, start exercising 10 to 15 minutes a day, five days a week, and work at it until it becomes routine and comfortable. Don't start by exercising 60 minutes each day, as this may be overwhelming and will end up becoming discouraging. Remember: Small, consistent changes over time will be manageable and rewarding.

Healthy Behaviors Goals

Now it's time to find a new behavior to turn into a habit. Talk with your family to decide on some goals you think you can reach successfully to start with. Here are some examples of goals to help you get started.

FAMILY GOALS

	Family	Adults	Child 1	Child 2
Parenting Goal Specific goal: Measure: Time frame:				
Healthy Behaviors Goal Specific goal: Measure: Time frame:		I will buy healthy cereal bars and water or sugar-free drinks for all of my children to eat next week I will go to the grocery store on Wednesday		I will drink a sugar-free drink and eat a cereal bar at least 3 times this week for breakfast on the way to school
Healthy Food Goal Specific goal: Measure: Time frame:				
Fitness Goal Specific goal: Measure: Time frame:				

Go to Appendix A for a full-size copy.

Fiction: What's the point of losing weight? The damage to my body is already done.

Fact: Losing a small amount of weight, in the range of approximately 15 percent, is frequently enough to reverse the symptoms associated with many obesity-related conditions. The liver can repair itself, and sugar metabolism (diabetes) and hypertension can normalize but frequently not be reversed if allowed to persist too long. The body can and will heal itself when helped along by weight loss!

3

• • •

Healthy Food Choices

You've heard the old saying "You are what you eat." Well, if you want to be healthy, then one of the most important things to do is eat healthy food and provide healthy food choices for your family. The challenge is to eat the right balance of foods so that everyone gets all the nutrients they need, select the healthier foods in each food group, and make sure each person is eating foods in the right portion size for their age. To assess how far along the ROAD to success you and your family are, answer the following questions.

Where Are You on the ROAD to Nutrition Savvy?

YES NO   *Check YES or NO to answer the following questions:*

☐   ☐   Does your family eat at least six servings from the bread, cereal, rice, and pasta group every day?

☐   ☐   Do you include several servings of whole-grain foods like whole wheat bread, oatmeal or whole-grain cereals, whole wheat crackers, and brown rice in your daily meals?

☐   ☐   Does your family eat at least three servings from the vegetable group every day?

☐   ☐   Does your family eat at least two servings from the fruit group every day?

☐   ☐   Do you purchase lower-fat products like low-fat sour cream or baked chips to help limit fat consumption in your family?

☐   ☐   Do you practice portion control when it comes to snacks and high-fat foods?

☐   ☐   Do you prepare your food using mostly low-fat cooking methods like grilling, broiling, baking, or stir-frying?

☐   ☐   Are you aware of the amount of soft drinks you consume and taking steps to limit the amounts?

☐   ☐   Are you aware of the amount of sweets your family eats and taking steps to offer healthy choices more often?

☐ ☐ Are you aware of the amount of juice your children drink every day?

☐ ☐ Do you eat meals prepared at home instead of going out to eat most evenings?

☐ ☐ Do you read nutrition labels when you shop so you can monitor the fat calories in the food you buy?

_____ *How many yes answers did you have?*

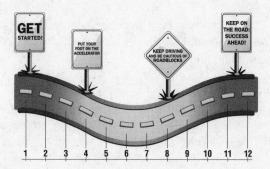

If you scored between 1 and 4, it is time to get your foot on the accelerator and focus on those small changes. If you scored between 5 and 8, you are on the ROAD to better nutrition, but watch out for those roadblocks. If you scored between 9 and 12, use the tips in this chapter to refine and improve your goals or decisions.

What Is a Healthy Diet?

A great way to start learning about a healthy diet is to look at the Food Guide Pyramid. The pyramid emphasizes six main food groups.

Food Guide Pyramid

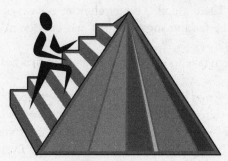

Grains
Meat and poultry
Dairy
Fruits
Vegetables
Oils

Source: www.mypyramid.gov.

A well-balanced diet incorporates foods from each of the food groups and even has a place for discretionary calories such as those from sweets, if used in moderation. It emphasizes fruits, vegetables, whole grains, and fat-free or low-fat milk and milk products; includes lean meats, poultry, fish, beans, eggs, and nuts; and is low in saturated fats, trans fats, cholesterol, salt, and added sugars.

Each of the food groups provides essential vitamins and minerals as well as protein or energy for a healthy body.

What Is Protein?

Protein supplies amino acids, which build, repair, and maintain body tissues like muscles. Protein provides 4 calories per gram. Protein-containing foods include eggs, meat, milk, and beans.

What Are Carbohydrates?

Carbohydrates are your body's main source of energy. They are either complex carbohydrates or starches like wild rice, potatoes, whole grains, or simple sugars. They provide 4 calories per gram.

What Are Fats?

Fats supply energy too, but also transport nutrients and are used by your cells. All fats provide 9 calories per gram, double the amount from other nutrients. That is why too much can quickly cause weight gain.

What Are Calories?

Calories are required for energy for your body and can come only from the foods you eat. However, eating too many calories each day can cause weight gain. The calories you eat need to be balanced with the calories you use in your daily activities and exercise. Eating only 100 more calories a day than you need can cause you to gain about a pound in one month. That is about 10 pounds in one year! Balance your calorie intake with your activity to maintain your weight; eat fewer calories or increase your activity to lose weight.

Your challenge is to pick foods from each of the food groups in their right proportion and serving size. There are also better choices in each of the food groups that help you watch the fat and sugar content and provide needed nutrients like fiber.

Here are some steps you can take to provide your family with a healthy diet.

- *Fruits:* Eat a variety of fruits to get the vitamins and minerals they provide. They can be fresh, canned, or dried. Two to four servings a day are enough for most people, but limit your choices from fruit juices, as they can fill you up and add lots of calories. Everyone should get at least one serving of a vitamin-C-rich food a day. Fruit is one of the easiest ways to get vitamin C in your diet, and it comes from sources like citrus fruits such as oranges or grapefruit, strawberries, guava, and papaya.

• *Vegetables:* Vegetables are a great source of vitamins and fiber. Try to eat three to five servings of vegetables a day. Dark green vegetables like broccoli and orange vegetables like carrots are great finger foods for kids. They are also high in vitamin A, which you should eat at least once every other day.

▶ HELPFUL HINT: **Vital Vegetable Vitamins**
There is a wide variation among vegetables in the amount of vitamins destroyed by cooking and it depends in part on the age, surface area (leafy or round), and cooking method. In general, the less time a vegetable or fruit is exposed to air, heat, and water, the more the vitamins are preserved. The nutrient retention is highest in foods cooked by microwave steaming, followed by microwave boiling, followed by steaming, and then by boiling.

• *Calcium-rich foods*: Fat-free or low-fat dairy products like milk, cheese, and yogurt are important in the diet to provide a good source of calcium. Try to get three to four servings a day of milk products or other calcium-fortified foods.

• *Whole grains*: Whole grains contain all the nutrients and fiber in the grain and are a good source of carbohydrates, which provide energy. Half of your daily grain choices should be whole grains. These can include whole wheat bread, whole-grain breakfast cereals, oats, and cornmeal.

• *Lean protein:* Choose lean meats like skinless poultry and fish to get the protein you need to build muscles and other body tissues. Keep it lean by baking, broiling, or grilling meats instead of frying. Peas, beans, nuts, and seeds are also good sources of protein and add variety to your diet.

What Should Be Limited in Most Diets?

• *Salt:* Most processed foods like frozen dinners and fast foods include a great quantity of salt. Fresher foods like lean meats and fruits and vegetables are much lower in salt. Minimize the amount of salt you add to foods when you cook or are at the table. Although salt has no calories, you should try to eat less than one teaspoon per day.

• *Sugar:* Sugar adds calories to the diet without adding any nutrients. Sugar is added to processed foods, sodas, fruit beverages, and cereals.

There is a lot of sugar in baked goods such as cookies, cake, and of course candy. Foods high in sugar should be limited to about one serving per day.

* *Fats:* While some fat is required for good health, some fat choices are better than others. Choose unsaturated fats like vegetable oils and avoid solid shortenings and margarines. Animal fats like butter and lard contain saturated fats and cholesterol and should be avoided. Try to limit fats in your diet to one to two tablespoons of fat or oil each day added to the foods you are eating since many foods also contain fat.

So, does your family eat the right number of foods from the pyramid? Here is a fun activity to see just how well everyone is doing. Have everyone write down everything they eat in one day. Now complete the Pyramid Work Sheet in Appendix A. Do the math. Are you over or under the target number of servings? Now each person has a good idea of what kinds of foods to add or subtract from their diet.

PLAN FOR YOUR YOUNG CHILD

Activity or Food Group	Recommended Amount	Total Amount of Activity or Servings Today	Difference: Amount Over or Under
Exercise	60 minutes		
Grains	6 oz		
Vegetables	2½ cups		
Fruits	2 cups		
Fats	Rarely or none		
Milk	3 cups		
Meat & Beans	5½ oz		

PORTION SIZES

Food Group	1 Serving =
Grains	1 slice bread 1 cup ready-to-eat cereal ½ cup cooked rice, pasta, or cereal

(continued)

PORTION SIZES (*continued*)

Food Group	1 Serving =
Vegetables	1 cup raw or cooked vegetables 1 cup vegetable juice 2 cups raw leafy greens
Fruits	1 cup fresh fruit 1 cup 100% fruit juice ½ cup dried fruit
Dairy	1 cup milk or yogurt 1½ oz natural cheese 2 oz processed cheese
Meat and Beans	1 oz meat, poultry, or fish ¼ cup cooked dry beans 1 egg 1 tablespoon peanut butter ½ oz nuts or seeds

▶ ROADBLOCK: Super-Size or Right Size
Learning what a proper portion size is can be challenging with so many large servings around us. Post the handy Food Group Portion Sizes chart in Appendix B that shows portions using simple household objects on your refrigerator!

Charting Your Favorite Foods

Now that you know what and how much of each of the food groups you and your children eat, let's explore each person's favorite foods in each group. Use this as a starting point to look closely at everyone's food choices. At the end of this chapter you will have another activity that can help find alternatives to some of these favorite foods—especially the ones that are full of fat and sugar.

Making Better Food Choices

It starts at the store. Remember that as the parent, you are in charge of what food comes into your home and you can say no to unhealthy foods.

▶ ROADBLOCK: Temptations at the Grocery Store
Shopping when you are hungry or with no real plan in mind results in buying many extra items. To avoid impulse buying, organize a

CHARTING FAVORITE FOODS

Type of Food	Favorite Dish or Way of Preparing Food
Vegetables	Creamed asparagus
	Boiled carrots
	Celery with salad dressing
	Green beans made with ham
	Broccoli with gooey cheese sauce

Write at least four to five favorite foods for each food group.

Type of Food	Favorite Dish or Way of Preparing Food
Vegetables	
Fruit	
Meat, beans, and other proteins	
Dairy	
Grains	
Fats and others (Include desserts and other foods here too!)	

shopping list before you go. Try using the Healthy Shopping List found in Appendix B the next time you go to the grocery store.

Here are some general shopping guidelines to help you choose the best foods.

- Fresh foods are mostly found on the outside aisles of the grocery store. Concentrate your shopping around the perimeter of the store instead of in the middle aisles where the more processed foods are located.
- Processed foods do save time. If you have a busy schedule, combine processed foods with fresh foods. Buy pregrilled chicken breast and make a fresh salad, or use frozen vegetables and bake a fresh fish fillet.
- Eat before you go to the grocery store. If you are hungry, you may be tempted to choose quick, high-fat snacks like chips or candy.

- Make a list before you shop. If you plan meals, you will not be as tempted to buy a lot of extras. Be flexible, however; if there are no green beans, for example, substitute another vegetable.
- Be firm about an established set of shopping rules. You don't want your children making a scene about an item you are unwilling to buy. Let them know ahead of time what is acceptable and what you are willing to be flexible about. For example, they may get to pick one snack item, but all cereals must be whole grain and low sugar.
- Try one new food item each week. Prepare "safe" meat and starch that everyone likes, but add a new vegetable. Not everyone will like each new thing, but keep trying.
- Save money by avoiding high-calorie, low-nutrient items like soda, fruit-flavored beverages, candy, chips, and high-sugar cereals.
- Individual packages of chips or cookies may be more expensive but may help your family control calories. Another tip is to portion your foods before you put them away. Purchase snack-size baggies and portion the snack foods into single-size portions. This helps to avoid excessive servings for the whole family.
- Give older kids items to find for you. Including them in the shopping may help encourage them to eat the meals prepared from those items as well as to read labels.
- Speaking of labels, one of the most important things you can do when shopping is to learn how to read a nutrition label. It gives you important information when comparing brands, or making healthier choices.

Reading Nutrition Labels

Everyone has seen the "Nutrition Facts" food label on packaged foods. You know it provides information about the nutrients in food, but actually reading all those hieroglyphics is another story—until you learn how to decipher the code.

The information found on food labels is based on general guidelines for an average diet of 2,000 calories per day—what an adult typically needs. Actual caloric and nutritional requirements vary by age, weight, gender, and activity levels.

Learning Label Language

To better understand the label, look at each section and the information it provides.

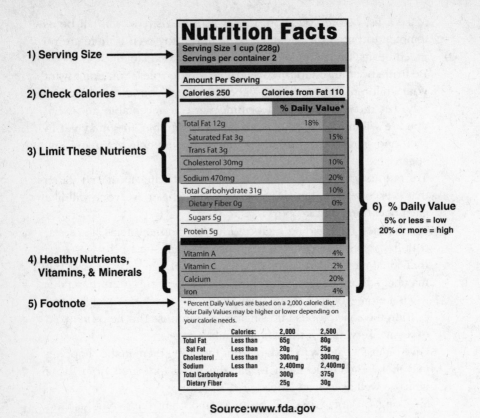

1) Serving Size

2) Check Calories

3) Limit These Nutrients

4) Healthy Nutrients, Vitamins, & Minerals

5) Footnote

6) % Daily Value
5% or less = low
20% or more = high

Nutrition Facts

Serving Size 1 cup (228g)
Servings per container 2

Amount Per Serving

Calories 250   Calories from Fat 110

	% Daily Value*
Total Fat 12g	18%
Saturated Fat 3g	15%
Trans Fat 3g	
Cholesterol 30mg	10%
Sodium 470mg	20%
Total Carbohydrate 31g	10%
Dietary Fiber 0g	0%
Sugars 5g	
Protein 5g	

Vitamin A	4%
Vitamin C	2%
Calcium	20%
Iron	4%

* Percent Daily Values are based on a 2,000 calorie diet.
Your Daily Values may be higher or lower depending on
your calorie needs.

	Calories:	2,000	2,500
Total Fat	Less than	65g	80g
Sat Fat	Less than	20g	25g
Cholesterol	Less than	300mg	300mg
Sodium	Less than	2,400mg	2,400mg
Total Carbohydrates		300g	375g
Dietary Fiber		25g	30g

Source:www.fda.gov

I. Serving Size

The nutrition label always lists a serving size. The serving size is an amount of food, such as cups, number of pieces, or number of grams. *Serving sizes help you understand how much you are eating.* In the sample label, one serving of macaroni and cheese equals 1 cup. If you ate the whole package, you would eat 2 cups. That doubles the calories and other nutrient numbers, including the % daily values.

Serving Size 1 cup (228g)
Servings per container 2

2. Check Calories

Amount Per Serving

Calories 250   Calories from Fat 110

The number of calories in a single serving is listed at the top left of the nutrition label. Calories are a measure of how much energy you get from a serving of this food. The calorie section of the label can help you manage your weight (gain, lose, or maintain). Remember: *The number of servings you consumes determines the number of calories you actually eat (your portion amount). Eating too many calories per day can lead to weight gain and obesity.* Another important part of the label, especially if you are limiting your fat intake, is the number of calories that come from fat. In this example, there are 250 calories in one serving of macaroni and cheese. Since there are 110 calories from fat in one serving, almost half of the calories in a single serving come from fat. This is one indication that one serving of macaroni and cheese is a moderately high-fat food choice.

3. Limit These Nutrients

	% Daily Value*
Total Fat 12g	18%
Saturated Fat 3g	15%
Trans Fat 3g	
Cholesterol 30mg	10%
Sodium 470mg	20%
Total Carbohydrate 31g	10%

These are nutrients people generally eat too much of. *Eating extra fat, saturated fat, trans fat, cholesterol, or sodium may increase your risk of certain chronic diseases such as heart disease, some cancers, and high blood pressure.* Important: Health experts recommend that you eat as little saturated fat, trans fat, and cholesterol as possible to have a nutritionally balanced diet.

4. Healthy Nutrients, Vitamins, & Minerals

Dietary Fiber 0g	0%
Sugars 5g	
Protein 5g	
Vitamin A	4%
Vitamin C	2%
Calcium	20%
Iron	4%

Most people do not get enough dietary fiber, vitamin A, vitamin C, calcium, and iron. *Eating plenty of these nutrients can improve your health and help reduce the risk of some diseases and conditions.* For example, getting enough calcium may reduce the risk of osteoporosis, a condition that results in brittle bones as one ages. Eating foods high in dietary fiber, such as whole grains, fruits, and vegetables, promotes healthy bowel function. A diet rich in soluble fiber and low in saturated fat and cholesterol may reduce the risk of heart disease.

5. Footnote

* Percent Daily Values are based on a 2,000 calorie diet. Your Daily Values may be higher or lower depending on your calorie needs.

	Calories:	2,000	2,500
Total Fat	Less than	65g	80g
Sat Fat	Less than	20g	25g
Cholesterol	Less than	300mg	300mg
Sodium	Less than	2,400mg	2,400mg
Total Carbohydrates		300g	375g
Dietary Fiber		25g	30g

The percentages on food labels are based on the recommended daily allowance (RDA). *This is the amount of a nutrient an adult should get each day.* Children may need less than 2,000 calories, and adolescents may need more than 2,500 calories. This footnote does not change from food item to food item, because it shows advice for the general population, not your personal calorie needs.

6. % Daily Value

% Daily Value*
18%
15%
10%
20%
10%

The % daily value (% DV) is based on a 2,000-calorie diet. The % DV *must* be on all food labels. In this case it shows that one serving of macaroni and cheese, which is 1 cup, provides 12 grams of fat. The recommended daily amount for a 2,000-calorie diet is less than 65 grams according to the footnote. One serving of macaroni and cheese provides 18 percent of that RDA. This guide also tells you that 5% DV or less is low for all nutrients. Similarly, 20% DV or more is high for all nutrients. In our example, 1 cup or one serving of macaroni and cheese is not considered "high fat" because it is below 20% DV. Since 18% is close to 20%, this may be considered a moderately high-fat food choice for one serving, or 1 cup. However, if you had 2 cups, or two servings, of macaroni and cheese, that would be 36% DV and thus a "high-fat" selection.

Preparing Healthy Meals

Parents are usually the ones who prepare food for the family (unless their children are old enough to help with food preparation). This means you are responsible for selecting healthy cooking methods, such as grilling, steaming, baking, or sautéing instead of frying. You can also use creative ways to add valuable nutrients to meals. Here are some ideas to introduce new foods, increase nutrients, and lower fats and calories in your meals:

Salads

- For nutrients and variety, add chopped apples, raisins, kiwi, or orange sections to green salads.
- Salads are a good filler and add lots of color to your plate. Use different vegetables in addition to different kinds of lettuce. Try mushrooms, different color bell peppers, carrots, radishes, spinach, cauliflower or broccoli florets, purple cabbage, green or snow peas, sliced onion, cucumber, or summer squash slices. Pick one or two per week to avoid spoilage.
- Shredded vegetable salads are easy for kids to chew, and older children can help by using a grater to shred the vegetables. Carrot raisin is a favorite shredded salad, but be careful not to add too much fat in the dressing.
- Citrus juice like lemon or orange with a little oil makes a quick and easy salad dressing.
- Choose low-fat or fat-free salad dressings. You can also add more vinegar and water to a regular dressing to reduce the proportion of fat.

Soups

- Combine a vegetable or lettuce salad with a meat- or fish-based soup for a complete meal.
- Use whole wheat noodles or other pasta or brown rice in soups.

- Bean-based soups like split pea or black bean are a good source of protein, or you can add beans to your favorite broth-based soup.
- Puree vegetables to use as a thickener in broth soups.

Breads and Starches

- Just because a bread is brown in color does not guarantee it is made with whole grains. Always read the label to make sure the word *whole* is listed first in the ingredient list, such as whole wheat or whole grain.
- Quick breads are a great place to hide shredded or pureed vegetables and fruits. Pumpkin, carrot, zucchini, banana, and apple all make good breads.
- Other additions to breads can include chopped fruits, nuts, or shredded low-fat cheese.

Nutrition Tip
You can substitute unsaturated oils like canola, walnut, or almond for half the butter or shortening in the quick breads.

- Cornmeal is a versatile whole grain. It can be made into corn bread, pancakes, polenta, and tamale pie–type casseroles.
- Toppings for pancakes can be pureed fruit instead of butter and syrup.
- Use corn tortillas or whole wheat pitas as alternatives to other breads.

Eggs and Dairy

- Some cheeses are very high in fat. Look for low-fat ricotta, part skim mozzarella, string cheese, or other varieties of reduced-fat products. You can also use a smaller amount of a stronger cheese to get the flavor without the calories. For example, instead of 1 cup of Colby cheese for a casserole, use ¼ cup of sharp cheddar.
- Substitute fat-free yogurt for sour cream or mayonnaise in a casserole or salad dressing. If the yogurt taste is too sour, mix it with fat-free ricotta cheese.
- Replace whole milk with skim milk.

Meats/Poultry/Fish

- Choose beef and pork cuts that have no visible fat, or remove the fat. Good choices are round steak, tenderloin, and 90 percent lean ground beef. Pork selections include trimmed loin chops and tenderloin.

Because there is very little waste with these cuts, you can use smaller portions.

- Add vegetables to meat dishes when possible: beef and peppers, beef stew, pot roast with vegetables, corned beef with cabbage, pork with apples, pork fried rice with bean sprouts or water chestnuts, meat loaf, and so on.
- Hot dogs and luncheon meats can be very high in fat (and sodium). Look for lower-fat or fat-free versions of those items.
- Turkey and chicken with the skin removed are among the leanest protein sources. Cooking with the skin adds fat to the final product.
- Fish can be baked, broiled, or poached in a low-fat liquid. Avoid deep-frying fish, but oven frying works well for fish fillets.

Fruits and Vegetables

- Fruits and vegetables must be available and accessible. Just buying them whole and putting them in the refrigerator is not enough to get your family to eat them. Foods that are washed, cut up, peeled, or cooked are easier for children to eat. Fill a container with baby carrots, celery sticks, broccoli florets, and cherry tomatoes and another container with dip. Place them in the front of the refrigerator for easy snacking. Grapes and strawberries are easy to clean and serve. Apple or pear slices turn brown after they are cut; soak them in a little lemon or pineapple juice in water to prevent browning. Peel and chunk a whole watermelon or cantaloupe. Peel oranges and make a container of sections for easy snacking.
- Try your favorite meat seasonings on vegetables: creole, curry, cumin, chili powder, mustard, or garlic.
- Cook vegetables in chicken broth instead of water for an enhanced flavor.
- If you don't have time to cut up fruits and vegetables, buy bag salads and get your toppings from the salad bar. Leave behind the high-fat croutons, cheese, and dressings.

Desserts

- Serve fresh fruits or sugar-free gelatin for dessert instead of other higher-calorie foods.
- Angel food cake is a good low-fat substitute for butter-type cakes.
- Puddings made with skim milk can be a good dessert and a source of calcium.
- Use fat-free whipped topping instead of whipped cream.

- Baked apples or peaches for dessert add a fruit serving to your meal.
- Make cookies with whole grains like oatmeal and whole wheat flour and add nuts and dried fruits like raisins or dates. Be sure to use oils for part of the fat.

Natural Weight Control

One strategy for promoting healthy eating behaviors is to avoid feeling hungry between meals. Nature provides us with foods that can promote that fullness but not add excessive calories. Foods that are high in fiber and water help you feel full yet reduce the calorie level of the meal. The idea is to eat a satisfying amount of food at a meal by consuming foods that provide fewer calories but fill a larger space in the stomach and leave you feeling full. For example: 100 calories = ½ cup raisins or 1⅔ cups grapes. As you can imagine, the larger volume of grapes is more filling than the small portion of dried fruit, yet the calories are the same.

High-fiber, filling foods include fresh fruits and vegetables, low-fat milk, cooked whole grains, beans, and broth-based soups. Foods with a lot of calories that take up little space in the stomach include high-fat foods such as cookies, chips, crackers, nutrient-dense nutrition bars, butter, deep-fat-fried items, sweets, and fats added at the table (butter, creams, gravy, cream-based sauces).

INSTEAD OF	TRY
Doughnut	Oatmeal with fruit
Chicken enchilada	Green salad with grilled chicken
Candy bar	6 ounces low-fat yogurt with ½ cup fresh fruit

Five Tips for Mealtime Success

Establish food rules to help make mealtime more successful:

1. Eat as a family as often as possible; make it a priority. If family dinner does not work for your family, try eating breakfast or lunch together. Remember to eat at the kitchen or dining room table, not in front of the television.
2. Don't focus on food! Avoid unpleasant food battles or nutrition lectures to your children during mealtime. Create an enjoyable environment by discussing positive topics, such as fun weekend plans or upcoming events at school.

3. Do not allow "special orders." Your kitchen is not a restaurant, so avoid serving your children different meals from the rest of the family. Instead, try to involve everyone in the meal-planning process and work together to prepare main dishes and side items that all agree on.

4. Model filling up on low-calorie fibrous foods (fruits, vegetables, and salads) before eating meat and starchy foods. This promotes fullness and reduces filling up on higher-calorie foods. Drink water throughout the meal as well.

5. Discourage "speed eating." Mealtime is not a race. Teach your children to enjoy mealtimes by eating small bites and engaging in the conversation.

Portion Control: Right-Sizing Your Foods

According to experts, one of Americans' biggest problems when it comes to controlling weight is portion size. In recent years, restaurants have tended to pile more and more food on each plate (or into each package), making huge portions seem run-of-the-mill.

PORTIONS

Food Groups (servings per day)	Age (years)					
	2–3	4–8	9–13 Females	Males	14–18 Females	Males
Grains: Bread, cereal, rice, pasta	3–5 oz	4–5 oz	5 oz	6 oz	6 oz	7 oz
Vegetables	1–1½ cup	1½–2½ cups	2 cups	2½ cups	2½ cups	3 cups
Fruits	1–1½ cup	1–1½ cups	1½ cups	1½ cups	1½ cups	2 cups
Meat, fish, beans, nuts	2–4 oz	3–5 oz	5 oz	5 oz	5 oz	6 oz
Dairy: milk, cheese, yogurt	2 cups	2–3 cups	3 cups	3 cups	3 cups	3 cups
Fats, oils, sweets*	——	——	——	——	——	——

*Follow these guidelines:

- Limit the amount of sugar your children get from candy sweets, juices, and other snacks.
- Limit fats like butter, shortening, and margarine, which contain more saturated and trans fats. (See Nutrition Glossary for a description of types of fats.)
- Do not restrict fats in children under age 2. The brain and other organs of young children need a certain amount of fat for proper development.

It is important to identify what makes appropriate portion sizes for your family. The portion sizes change as your children grow and are different for boys and girls.

The brief summary at the bottom of the preceding page recommends portion sizes for each food category per day.

Are All Fats Created Equal?

Although it may seem that eliminating fat or following a very low-fat diet will lead to fat loss, in fact, fats are essential to life and are used for multiple bodily functions. Fats are necessary for the absorption of fat-soluble vitamins (A, D, E, and K), which help with bone and tooth development, vision, and preventing blood clots and damage to cell membranes. Fats also serve as vital components of cell membranes, help make hormones, protect your organs, and are a great energy source. Finally, fats add flavor to foods, help keep you feeling full, and assist in keeping blood sugar levels stable. But not all fats are created equal.

Unsaturated Fats

Unsaturated fats are usually liquid at room temperature. They are found in most vegetable products, fish, and some oils. Unsaturated fats are classified as *monounsaturated,* such as canola and olive oil, and *polyunsaturated,* such as corn, safflower, sunflower, and fish oils.

Both types of unsaturated fat can be used in place of saturated fat in your diet, and they will help to lower cholesterol levels. However, all types of fats have 9 calories per gram and can to lead to weight gain when used in excess.

Saturated Fats

Saturated fats, known as the bad or unhealthy fats, are solid or mostly solid at room temperature. Saturated fats are primarily of animal origin, such as fats in the skin of meat and poultry and in dairy products (cheese, butter, lard, and milk). Saturated fats are also found in some vegetable oils (palm, palm kernel, and coconut oil). A diet high in saturated fats causes the body to make excess cholesterol, which increases the risk of heart disease.

Trans Fats

Trans fats are created from mostly unsaturated fats by making them more saturated through a process called *hydrogenation*. This process involves changing the chemical structure of unsaturated fats by adding hydrogen atoms. The purpose is to increase the shelf life of a product, which allows manufacturers to produce mass amounts of the product at one time, which lowers its cost.

As of January 1, 2006, manufacturers of conventional foods and some dietary supplements must list trans fats on the nutrition label under saturated fat. According to the Food and Drug Administration (FDA), scientists have established a relationship between trans fat consumption and an increased risk for heart disease. Therefore, adding this information to food labels is intended to make the public more aware of the amount of trans fats that may be hidden in products they consume.

The best way to evaluate a food product for trans fats is to review the nutrition label. If you see the words *hydrogenated* or *partially hydrogenated oils,* then the food contains trans fats. Foods that commonly contain trans fats include processed foods, margarines, shortenings, crackers, candy, baked goods, chips, snack foods, fried foods, condiments, and salad dressings. The good news is that many companies have worked to develop products that contain no trans fats, and this information is proudly displayed on many food labels.

Healthy New Changes in Many Snack Foods

- 100-calorie preportioned snack packages
- 3 grams of whole grain
- no artificial flavors
- zero grams of trans fat
- 3 grams of total fat with little or no saturated fat

How Much Fat Should My Child Consume?

For children older than two, the United States Department of Agriculture's (USDA) Dietary Guidelines for Americans, 2005, recommends the following:

- Consume less than 10 percent of calories from saturated fatty acids and fewer than 300 mg/day of cholesterol, and keep trans fatty acid consumption as low as possible.
- Keep total fat intake between 20 and 35 percent of calories, with most fats coming from sources of polyunsaturated and monounsaturated fatty acids, such as fish, nuts, and vegetable oils.
- When selecting meat, poultry, dry beans, and milk or milk products, choose lean, low-fat, or fat free.

Smarter Sugar Choices

Sugar is everywhere. Not only is it found in obvious foods and drinks such as sugary cereals, candy, cookies, and soda, but it is also hidden in many foods you might not be aware of. A few examples include cereal, cereal bars, crackers, ketchup, mayonnaise, pasta sauce, peanut butter, salad dressing, and marinades. Basically, most highly processed and prepackaged foods have a sugar sweetner added. An increasing percentage of added sweetner comes from corn syrup in the form of high-fructose corn syrup (HFCS). HFCS is only one of many sugars added to processed foods today.

Increase in Sugar Consumption

Between 1970 and 1990, the use of high-fructose corn syrup increased 1,000 percent, and individual consumption of HFCS rose from 0.5 pound to 62.4 pounds a year.

The challenge is that added sugar is not always obvious. Start scanning the ingredients of the foods and drinks you consume to see for yourself how many products contain a sugar filler! First, look at the difference between natural sugars and added sugars. Natural sugars are found in foods like fruits and dairy products. For example, a fresh apple has about 15 grams of sugar, and one cup of milk has 12 grams of sugar. These foods have no added sugar and both are considered healthy foods that are rich in many vitamins and minerals. A processed food such as a can of regular soda (12 ounces) contains 13 teaspoons of sugar in the form of HFCS—between 36 and 44 grams of total added sugar.

So how do you tell the difference between foods and drinks with natural sugar and those with added sugars? The nutrition label does not distinguish between natural and added sugars, so you must read the ingredients list on each product.

▶ ROADBLOCK: Look for Hidden Sugar

Here are some other forms of sugar to be aware of:

• raw sugar	• dextrose*
• sucrose*	• fructose*
• sugar	• fruit juice concentrates
• syrup	• glucose*
• brown sugar	• high-fructose corn syrup
• corn sweetener	• honey
• corn syrup	• invert sugar

- lactose*
- maltose*
- malt syrup
- molasses

*The suffix -*ose* always indicates sugar.

Remember that the ingredients are listed in order of greatest to least amount in the product. If sucrose (sugar) is the first ingredient listed, it means that sucrose is the main ingredient in the product.

Avoid or limit products that list added sugars high on the ingredient list. The 2005 USDA Dietary Guidelines suggest that Americans "choose and prepare foods and beverages with little added sugars or caloric sweeteners." The American Dietetic Association (ADA) advises to limit added sugars to less than 25 percent of daily calories.

▶ HELPFUL HINT: Try New Tastes at Least Ten Times

Research shows that children need to have several opportunities to taste something new before a preference "grows on them." According to studies, parents should keep trying between ten and fifteen times. After fifteen tries, it's likely that the child isn't going to change his or her mind at this point in time.

Creating Healthy Choices

Eating a healthy diet at school and at home increases your children's stamina and brainpower.

Ten year-old Molly loves milk. She knows that milk is rich in calcium, which helps her bones grow strong. However, Molly's doctor informed her at her yearly checkup that she is overweight. He suggested that Molly schedule an appointment with the clinic dietitian to discuss healthy eating habits. The dietitian recommended that one change Molly could make in her diet was to switch from whole milk to skim milk. Molly agreed to make this simple change.

Molly also decided to do some research on the differences between whole milk and skim. She went to the grocery store with her mother and together they read the nutrition labels on the milk cartons. Molly discovered that by switching to skim milk she would reduce her calory intake per cup of milk by 70 calories. Wow! She also noticed that the protein and calcium amounts were identical in whole milk, 2%, 1%, and skim milk. The only difference was the fat content.

Molly next calculated that she would actually save 210 calories per day since she drinks 3 cups of milk per day; this equals 1,470 calories per week, which amounts to about a ½-pound weight loss per week (3,500 calories=1 pound).

Molly decided that switching to skim milk was a very easy diet change she could make to help her lose weight.

Start with Breakfast

Breakfast is a problem for many families. Grabbing doughnuts or pastries or driving through the fast-food window on the way to school seems much easier than whipping up a healthy meal while trying to get everyone out the door to work and school.

Breakfast does not need to be a gourmet affair every day. Be creative. Try to include at least two or three different groups of food in the breakfast. For example, try one of these combinations:

- 1 frozen waffle, 1–2 tablespoons of peanut butter, and 1 cup of low-fat milk
- ¾ cup cornflakes, 1 cup of low-fat milk, and 1 banana
- 1 cup of oatmeal and ½ cup of unsweetened fruit cocktail

Try to make breakfast different each day. That way it is fun and exciting, and your children will never know what to expect—except something healthy and tasty.

▶ **HELPFUL HINT: Don't Dress Up Your Food**
Many foods can be healthy choices—until you start adding to them. Watch how you "dress up" a food. For example, an English muffin can be perfectly healthy, but if you drench it in butter—it quickly becomes *un*healthy.

More Yummy Breakfast Options

- oatmeal
- grits
- Cream of Wheat
- English muffin
- muffin (the muffin-pan size, not megasize)
- bagel (3-inch diameter, usually frozen) or ½ big bagel
- fruit smoothie (whole fruits, plain low-fat yogurt, and ice)
- whole-grain wheat toast
- whole fruit (keeps you fuller than fruit juice)
- tortilla wrap (veggies and egg whites or turkey and low-fat cheese)

- low-fat yogurt with granola on top
- reduced-fat peanut butter
- dry whole-grain cereal to go

Make Lunch Alluring

The school lunch program options have changed in recent years, so you may want to speak with your children's school food service manager to learn about healthy menu options. Each week you can review the week's menu with your children to help teach them how to select the most nutritious foods available.

Make lunch and snacks healthy—but keep them exciting too. Here is one idea to get you started: Send sandwiches or gelatin cutouts shaped with cookie cutters. This extra touch lets your children know that they are special.

Cruising Through the Alphabet of Healthy Snacks

Struggling with snack ideas? Here are a few to start with.

A Apples, applesauce, animal crackers, angel food cake

B Bananas, bran muffins, baked chips or crackers, bread sticks

C Crackers, cereal bars, cantaloupe slices, low-fat cheese cubes or sticks, carrot sticks

D Dried fruit, low-fat dip for raw vegetables

E Egg salad

F Fresh fruit, frozen fruit bars, frozen grapes

G Granola, grapes, grapefruit, graham crackers, gelatin

H Honeydew melon slices

I Ice cream (low-fat) or sherbet

J 100% fruit juice

K Kiwi, kebabs made from fruits and vegetables

L Lean meat on half a sandwich

M Muffins, minibagels

N Nectarines

O Oranges, oatmeal cookies

U Unsweetened canned fruits

P Peaches, plums, pumpkin bread, pretzels, popcorn (lite)

V Vanilla wafers, raw vegetables

Q Quiche (vegetable), quick breads, quench your thirst with water

W Watermelon triangles, whole wheat snack crackers

R Raisins, raspberries, rice cakes

X Extra-lean lunch meats

S Strawberries, string cheese

Y Yogurt (low-fat, no added sugar)

T Turkey or tuna sandwich, tomatoes

Z Zucchini bread

Don't Forget the Water

Water is an excellent way to stay hydrated. Adults can drink six to eight 8-ounce servings a day, although this much is probably not required. Fruits and vegetables are 80 to 90 percent water and can help you meet your water needs.

Regular sodas, juice drinks, and fruit punches contain more sugar than you need—approximately 100 calories for an 8-ounce serving. Juices that are 100-percent fruit juice contain vitamins, minerals, and fiber that your body needs, but in excess, they just provide unneeded calories. Limit all of these beverages to one serving a day, or skip them altogether. The American Academy of Pediatrics recommends allowing no more than two 4-ounce servings of juice a day. If you do choose them, be certain to select the healthier varieties.

Limit sports drinks for use during intense exercise or after prolonged exercise or lengthy exposure to outdoor heat (see page 166 in Chapter 9 for more details).

Low-Calorie Beverages
- water
- diet soda
- 1% milk
- skim milk
- diet fruit juices
- unsweetened tea

Eating Out and About*

In this fast-paced world, continuing to eat a healthy diet when always on the go is challenging. But making wise food choices—even on the run—helps you and your family continue on the ROAD to overall health and weight loss or maintenance.

In May 1997, the Food and Drug Administration made it mandatory that any restaurant claiming to have "heart healthy" or "low-fat" foods must be able to provide the consumer with nutritional information to support the claim. However, the nutritional information need not be presented within easy sight, as on processed and packaged foods. Instead, the restaurant can simply keep a binder with nutritional information on those particular foods.

Currently many nutrition bills are going through the legislative process. One would require restaurants belonging to a chain of twenty or more to post nutritional information next to the item on the menu or menu board. It would include total calories, grams of saturated and trans fats, and milligrams of sodium.

Many of the popular restaurants and fast-food chains have voluntarily put the nutritional information on the Web. By logging onto their Web sites, you can usually find the information fairly easily.

General Restaurant Tips

- If you know you are going to be eating out during the day, plan on eating healthier, lighter meals.
- Be prepared either to share an entrée with someone, or automatically ask for a "to-go" box when the food is brought. Cut everything on your plate in half and put one-half in the box for another meal.
- Think twice about all-you-can-eat buffets. Too many choices and waiting to get your money's worth of food usually result in a very high-calorie meal.
- Ask the waiter not to bring the premeal basket of bread or chips.
- Don't be afraid to ask how foods are cooked and to specify how you would like your food prepared.
- Ask for dressings and other sauces on the side.
- Choose fresh fruit for dessert.
- Eat slowly, so you have time to feel full and avoid overeating.
- Watch out for the sodas and sweet tea. Try unsweetened tea, diet soda, or, better yet, water.

*Adapted from the American Heart Association.

- Parents, limit your alcohol consumption. One ounce of alcohol typically contains about 84 calories, and that's without the added mix like soda.

Fast Food

Follow these tips for smart food choices:

- Avoid burgers with cheese, special sauce, mayonnaise, and bacon—they add more fat and calories.
- Pickles, onions, lettuce, tomato, mustard, and ketchup add flavor without adding fat.
- Avoid fried fish—that choice is often the highest-calorie food on the menu.
- Watch out for the "extra" words like *giant, deluxe, biggie-size, super-size,* and *jumbo.*
- A baked potato may be a healthy option, but not if it is topped with butter or sour cream.

INSTEAD OF	TRY
Danish, doughnut	English muffin or small bagel
Jumbo cheeseburger	Grilled chicken, sliced meats, or 2 oz hamburger such as a junior burger
Fried chicken or taco	Grilled chicken or salad bar (with lite dressing)
Fried chicken nuggets/strips	Chicken fajita pita
French fries	Small baked potato with vegetable or low-fat yogurt topping
Regular potato chips	Baked potato chips, pretzels
Milk shake	Fat-free milk, diet soda, water

American/Family Restaurants

Many options are available at these restaurants, so be sure to choose wisely! Don't be afraid to ask for something that is not listed on the menu exactly the way you want it.

Here are some more helpful hints:

- Avoid dishes with lots of cheese, sour cream, or mayonnaise.
- Salads make great meal choices, but be careful of the dressing. Ask

for lite or fat-free dressing on the side, so you can control how much you use. Watch extras that are added to the salad, such as cheese, croutons, eggs, and bacon.
- Watch out for portion sizes.

INSTEAD OF	TRY
Cream soup	Broth-based soup with vegetables
Fried oysters, seafood, or chicken	Boiled shrimp; baked, broiled, or grilled seafood or chicken
Buffalo chicken wings	Grilled chicken strips tossed in buffalo wing sauce
Main entrée	Side salad with a low-fat appetizer
Fried chicken sandwich	Grilled chicken sandwich
Cheeseburger	Hamburger or veggie burger
French fries	Baked potato, boiled potatoes, rice, cooked vegetables—with no added butter or oil
Hot fudge sundae or ice cream	Nonfat yogurt, sherbet, or fruit

Asian Food

Main-dish items are usually very large. Order with the idea that you are going to be sharing or taking home extra food.

- Stir-fried items are cooked using oil and salt. Ask for stir-fried dishes to be cooked using less oil.
- Choose entrées with lots of vegetables.
- Substitute chicken for duck, which is very fatty.
- Skip the crispy fried noodles on the table.

INSTEAD OF	TRY
Egg drop soup	Wonton or hot-and-sour soup
Egg rolls or fried wontons	Steamed dumplings
Fried entrées	Broiled, steamed, or lightly stir-fried vegetables

Dishes with fried meat	Dishes with lots of vegetables
Fried rice	Steamed white or brown rice

Greek or Middle Eastern Foods

People living in the Mediterranean have a diet that is lower in saturated and trans fats than that in the United States. You can follow their lead to eat more healthily:

- Ask for dishes to be prepared with less oil and for high-sodium foods (such as olives and feta cheese) to be served on the side.
- Ask for salad dressing and sauces on the side.
- Phyllo pastry dishes are usually very high in butter, so avoid them.
- Most Greek desserts are high in fat and sugar. If you splurge, plan to share with a friend.
- Use small amounts of feta cheese.
- Consider using hummus (made from chickpeas) instead of typical dressings.
- Eat a cucumber and tomato salad prior to the entrée.

INSTEAD OF	TRY
Fried calamari	Dolmas (rice mixture wrapped in grape leaves)
Moussaka (lamb and beef casserole)	Roast lamb, shish kebab (lots of red meat), or chicken kebab
Creamy or cheesy entrées	Couscous or bulgar wheat with vegetables or chicken
Gyro	Chicken pita sandwich
Baklava and other pastries	Fruit

Italian Food

Italian dishes tend to be made with cheese and heavy sauces. Here are some tips to lead to more healthy selections.

- Order dishes prepared with mushrooms, garlic, lemon, or marinara sauce.
- Avoid Parmesan cheese.
- Avoid entrées made with more than one cheese, such as four-cheese lasagna or three-cheese manicotti.

- If choosing pizza, avoid extra cheese, pepperoni, and sausage toppings, as well as stuffed crust pizza.
- Choose toppings like spinach, mushrooms, broccoli, and roasted peppers.

INSTEAD OF	TRY
Fried calamari	Roasted peppers or minestrone soup
Fried mozzarella	Bruschetta
Cheese- or meat-filled pastas	Pasta primavera (with sautéed garden vegetables)
Pasta with butter or cream sauces (e.g., Alfredo sauce)	Pasta with red or marinara sauce (tomatoes, onions, garlic)

Mexican Food

Mexican foods are characterized by high-fat items such as cheese, sour cream, and fried foods. Follow these tips for smarter food choices.

- To help limit your (fried) tortilla chip intake, put a small amount on your plate and then ask the waiter to take the basket away from the table.
- Use more salsa and lime for flavor, and limit sour cream and guacamole on the entrées.
- Avoid creamy or cheesy sauces.
- If you order taco salad, don't eat the fried shell and ask for dressing on the side.

INSTEAD OF	TRY
Flour torilla (may contain lard)	Corn tortilla (almost no fat)
Chalupa, taco	Taco salad or fajita salad (don't eat the shell)
Flauta, chimichanga, burrito	Chicken or beef enchilada with red sauce or salsa
Quesadilla	Fajita (grilled chicken with onions, diced tomatoes, lettuce; no sour cream or guacamole)
Refried beans	*Frijoles a la charra* (borracho beans)
Carnitas or chorizo (fried meat)	Grilled fish or chicken breast

Indian Food

Indian dishes tend to contain more vegetables and carbohydrates and less meat and protein. They frequently use legumes, such as lentils, which contain a high amount of protein. Avoid foods that are fried or sautéed in ghee, a clarified butter. Sesame and coconut oils are the most frequently used oils. Here are some tips for making Indian food extra-healthy:

* Start with a salad or yogurt with chopped or shredded vegetables.
* Choose chicken or seafood rather than beef or lamb.
* Choose dishes with little or no ghee.
* Order one protein and one vegetable dish to cut down on fat and calories.

INSTEAD OF	TRY
Samosa (fried, stuffed vegetable turnover)	Papadum or papad (crispy thin lentil wafers)
Korma (meat with rich yogurt sauce)	Chicken or beef tikka (roasted in an oven with mild spices) or chicken or beef tandoori (marinated in spices, baked)
Curry made with coconut milk or cream	Curry with a vegetable or dal base
Pakora (deep-fried dough with vegetables)	*Gobhi matar tamatar* (cauliflower with peas and tomatoes)
Sauced rice	Fragrant steamed rice
Fried or stuffed bread	Chapati (thin, dry whole wheat bread), naan (leavened bread, baked with poppyseeds)

Cajun Food

Cajun dishes are usually spicy and contain high-fat ingredients, but most of them can be made with less fat. Follow these tips:

* Avoid fried seafood and hush puppies.
* Blackened entrées are usually dipped in butter or oil, covered with spices, and panfried. Ask for them to be grilled instead, using the same spices.

- Ask for food items to be cooked in less oil.
- Ask for all sauces and gravies on the side.

INSTEAD OF	TRY
Fried crawfish or shrimp	Boiled crawfish or shrimp
Gumbo, étouffée, and sauces made with roux (butter and flour)	Creole and jambalaya dishes
Fried seafood	Broiled, baked, or grilled seafood
Dirty rice	Steamed white or brown rice
Red beans and rice with sausage	Red beans and rice with no sausage
Fried shrimp po'boy	Turkey or roast beef poboy sandwich

▶ **ROADBLOCK: Ideas for Eating on the Road**
When you know that you and your family are going to be in a hurry, consider packing food to take with you in the car instead of eating fast food. This also is convenient for snacktimes and activities before and after school.

- whole-grain bread or bagels
- small cans of water-packed tuna
- fresh veggies, like baby carrots or carrot and celery sticks
- fresh fruits such as bananas, apples, pears, oranges, and nectarines
- small fruit cups packed in lite syrup
- dried fruits such as raisins, figs, and apricots
- low-fat yogurt (must be kept in cooler on ice)
- homemade low-fat whole-grain muffins or quick breads (pumpkin, banana)
- air-popped popcorn (no butter)
- low-fat whole-grain crackers or pretzels
- string mozzarella cheese (must be kept in cooler on ice)
- dry-roasted, lightly salted nuts
- dry whole-grain cereals
- ½ peanut butter sandwich on whole wheat bread
- water
- unsweetened iced tea

New Favorite Foods

Now that you understand more about nutrition and healthy options, revisit the list you made at the beginning of the chapter in "Charting Favorite Foods."

Use the new list (below) to help you and your children name healthier alternatives for favorite foods. For example, if one of the favorite foods is ice cream, a new favorite food could be low-fat frozen yogurt. If the favorite food was fried chicken, a new favorite food could be baked chicken with no skin.

NEW FAVORITE FOODS

Type of Food	Favorite Dish or Way of Preparing Food	Healthier Version
Vegetables		
Fruit		
Meat, beans, and other proteins		
Dairy		
Grains		
Fats and others (Include desserts and other foods here too!)		

Now that you have a list of new favorite foods, challenge yourself and your family to try at least one of these new foods each day. Try a particular dish or vegetable several times, experimenting with different seasonings. For example, you could have dill carrots, cinnamon carrots, ginger carrots, or garlic carrots. Be creative and the possibilities are limitless!

Setting Goals for Choosing Healthier Foods

Now that you have assessed your and your family's diet, learned about healthy food choices, and identified some new ones to try, it's time to set some goals specific to food choices.

Write one or two goals centered around healthier food choices. Here is an example to get you started:

FAMILY GOALS

	Family	Adults	Child 1	Child 2
Parenting Goal Specific goal: Measure: Time frame:				
Healthy Behaviors Goal Specific goal: Measure: Time frame:				
Healthy Food Goal Specific goal: Measure: Time frame:		I will prepare a vegetable for dinner Every night this week Tuesday will be broccoli night	I'm going to try broccoli Two bites At dinnner	
Fitness Goal Specific goal: Measure: Time frame:				

Go to Appendix A for a full-size copy.

Fiction: I just drink soft drinks to quench my thirst. It's only liquid—I shouldn't gain weight from that.

Fact: Many soft drinks and juices contain sugar, which does contain calories—about 150 in one 12-ounce can of soda. The average person needs to exercise 30 to 60 minutes to burn off that many calories.

4

• • •

Making Fitness Fun
and Effective

Research over the years has demonstrated that physical activity is a contributing factor to weight loss, just as inactivity is a factor in being overweight. Healthy eating habits and physical activity are both important for a successful weight-loss program. The goal is to use up more energy with exercise than you take in with food. Effective exercise is regular, consistent, and incorporated into daily life.

Hey, parents, take this quick quiz to get a better sense of where you and your children are at when it comes to fitness.

Where Are You on the ROAD to Fitness Readiness?

YES NO *Check YES or NO to answer the following questions:*

☐ ☐ Can you think of three activities that you enjoy doing?

☐ ☐ Can you think of three activities that your children enjoy doing?

☐ ☐ Can you think of three activities that you and your children can do together?

☐ ☐ Do you walk to school or to do errands?

☐ ☐ Do you have athletic shoes and loose clothing for activity/exercise?

☐ ☐ Do you exercise at least three times a week?

☐ ☐ Do you usually remember to warm up and cool down with exercise?

☐ ☐ Do you know when *not* to exercise?

☐ ☐ Can you tell if you are getting enough activity/exercise?

☐ ☐ Do all members of your family get regular activity/exercise?

☐ ☐ Do you try new types of activity/exercise at least once a month?

☐ ☐ Do you have goals for getting regular activity/exercise?

_____ *How many yes answers did you have?*

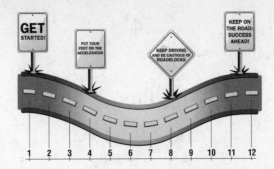

If you scored between 1 and 4, it is time to get your foot on the accelerator and focus on getting your family moving. If you scored between 5 and 8, you are on the ROAD to better health, but watch out for roadblocks that may interfere with your success. If you scored between 9 and 12, use the tips in this chapter to refine and improve your goals or decisions.

The Power of Movement

As an adult, you have probably noticed that you feel a little stiff when you get up after sitting for a long time. That's because your body wasn't designed to be inactive. You were designed for movement, such as walking, running, bending, climbing, swimming, and jumping. Unfortunately, our society has evolved in such a way that most people live in a more inactive state.

What was once done by manual labor is now done by machine. Schools and jobs require people to sit most of the day. To make up for that, people must consciously focus on increasing their activity level throughout the day to counterbalance sitting so much at home, work, and school.

Numerous benefits come from physical activity and exercise:

- Exercise helps keep the body working at its best.
- Certain types of activities (running, swimming, bicycling) increase the strength of the heart and lungs.
- Other activities (weight lifting) increase the strength of the muscles, which helps the body burn calories more efficiently.
- Exercise can help lower blood pressure and cholesterol, relieve stress, and reduce the risk of some types of cancer.
- Decreased weight comes from burning calories and fat.
- Endurance improves with more exercise.
- Energy levels improve with more exercise.
- Exercise can have a positive impact on various other health problems associated with being overweight, such as joint pain, diabetes, cardiac and respiratory conditions, sleep apnea, and others.

Additional benefits of exercise are psychological, such as an increase in your sense of well-being and self-worth, a decrease in stress, an increase in peer interaction, and an increase in family time.

Decrease in Activity Leads to Increase in Weight

Children and adolescents are spending less time being active, whether due to watching TV, playing video games, or spending time online. A study by William Dietz and Steven Gortmaker reports that children spend as much time watching TV as they do attending school.

The American Academy of Pediatrics recommends limiting "screen time" (including computers as well as video games and TV) to a maximum of 2 hours per day for children older than two years of age and no screen time for children under the age of two. The important thing to note is what children and adolescents are doing, or not doing, because of time spent in front of a television or video screen. One research study demonstrated that the body's metabolism slows down when watching TV to a rate that is actually lower than during rest. At the same time that metabolism decreases, TV viewing is often accompanied by snacking—typically with high-fat and high-sugar foods and beverages.

A study by Donna Matheson and colleagues demonstrated that television viewing influences the type and amount of foods consumed by children when watching TV. Children aged two to six years were shown a video of a popular cartoon with commercials embedded. Those exposed to the video with embedded commercials were more likely to choose the advertised items than children who saw the video without commercials. Just think how often children, even very young ones, know the words to commercial jingles.

The Centers for Disease Control conducted a Youth Risk Behavior Survey in 1990 of high school students from all fifty states and the District of Columbia. The results showed that the respondents who were classified as "low active" (fewer than two days of light exercise and no days of hard exercise in the past fourteen days) tended to be female, between the ages of sixteen and eighteen, and nonwhite. Lower physical activity was also associated with other risky health behaviors: cigarette smoking, poor dietary habits, increased TV viewing, and failure to wear a seat belt.

Exercise to Lose Weight

The words *physical activity* and *exercise* are often used interchangeably, but there is a difference between them. Physical activity is any type of movement, whereas exercise implies a specific activity done for a specific amount of time at a certain intensity. Both are beneficial and will burn calories and boost energy levels.

Exercise is an important key to long-term weight loss. It is often divided into two types: aerobic and anaerobic. *Aerobic* means "with oxygen" and involves the increased use of the lungs, heart, blood vessels, and large muscles in the process of transporting oxygen from the air we breathe to the muscles. Aerobic exercises, such as jogging, biking, and dancing, involve muscle groups used continuously for at least 15 to 20 minutes to allow the body to burn stored fat.

Anaerobic ("without oxygen") exercises, such as weight lifting, involve short bursts of intense activity. This movement challenges the muscles, making them stronger over time. In turn, the muscles improve posture, strengthen the muscles used for breathing, build stomach and back muscles (which decreases back pain), improve efficiency of movement, and make daily activities easier.

Getting Started

Do you find yourself getting bored or sleepy if you have to sit for more than 30 minutes doing the same thing? The reason for this is that concentration and performance typically decline after 30 minutes of intense mental activity. So for every 30 minutes that you sit, take a quick fitness break for about 3 to 5 minutes to recharge your battery and boost your energy level. Stretch or go for a short walk. Sitting burns 30 to 50 calories per hour, standing burns 60 to 110 calories per hour, and walking slowly burns 120 to 200 calories per hour.

Look at your daily routine, individually and as a family, to determine small ways that you can increase your activity levels. Consider these examples:

- If you sit when you talk on the phone, stand up or walk around instead.
- Instead of circling to find a parking space close to your destination, park farther away and walk there briskly.
- Take the stairs—up or down one flight at first, and switch to the elevator for the rest of the way if needed, until you build up your stamina.
- If you want something, get up and get it yourself instead of asking someone else to get it for you.

These changes may not sound like much, but every little bit over time makes a difference. People's most common pitfall when they set goals is that they aim too high too quickly and set themselves up for failure from the beginning. For example, if your goal was to run a marathon, you typically wouldn't get out of bed one day, head out the door, and run twenty-six miles. It takes months of training to gradually increase your stamina and the distance you run and to let your body adjust to the training regimen. The same idea holds true for any goal.

To get started, you must first determine what you want to achieve:

- What dietary changes need to occur?
- How much physical activity and exercise do you need to accomplish your goal of weight loss?
- Who can help? A critical step in trying to change lifestyle habits, in addition to establishing a plan of action, is to recruit help. Schedule ahead to work out with your friends or family members, or join a class or a team.

Another key to being successful with goal setting is to take small steps. Expecting to exercise every day, if it has been years since you last exercised, is probably not realistic. Start by taking a walk around your block every other day, and then add on from there.

The next step is to set up a plan for how to carry out that goal.

Decide What Works for You

You can choose more than one activity or exercise. Younger kids need more variety in their activities, while older kids tend to narrow down to one or two types, which helps them achieve a sense of accomplishment.

In addition to choosing an activity that is fun, try to pick one that's a challenge. This will help keep it interesting and enable you to see results as you make progress.

▶ ROADBLOCK: **What to Do on a Rainy Day!**
Don't let bad weather keep you from being active. Plan indoor activities such as dance videos, interactive games such as Twister, or have some fun with household chores. Remember, it's important to be consistent about being active, so keep inclement weather excuses to a minimum with alternate activities to choose from.

Fun Fitness Options

The list of fun fitness options can go on and on. There are no rules to limit what you can do to get up and get moving—as long as your environment is safe and your activities are enjoyable. Remember that younger children need a variety of activities to keep them interested, and their attention seems to stay focused best in short bouts.

Creativity is the key. An old mattress can be used as an indoor minitrampoline. A soft (Nerf type) basketball can be played with inside. Here are some more ideas:

- jump rope
- hula hoop
- Twister
- dance (or games like Dance Dance Revolution)
- musical chairs
- tag
- putt-putt golf
- roller-skating
- Rollerblading
- broom hockey
- rock climbing
- gardening

Think back to when you were a kid. What activities did you enjoy? Share them with your children and make it a family activity.

▶ HELPFUL HINT: **Pilates Pilot Proves Promising**
A 2005 pilot study conducted by the Children's Nutrition Research Center, Department of Pediatrics at Baylor College of Medicine, showed that girls who participated in a four-week Pilates class significantly lowered their BMI percentile while maintaining a high rate of enjoyment. Pilates holds promise as a means of reducing obesity, and further research is under way.

Plan as a Family

When planning for activity or exercise, involve the family. Friends are welcome too. Children are more motivated to participate in activities and exercise when family or friends are involved.

Approach fitness as a change in lifestyle—not just a temporary trial. Change your everyday routines. For instance, walk together to the mailbox, and have your children assist with chores like setting the table, cleaning the dishes, vacuuming, or mowing the lawn. Encourage your children to take care of their own belongings.

Children learn through example, so make sure they see you participating in activities with them. To help make sure that happens, set specific times for activity and exercise and make a schedule.

▶ HELPFUL HINT: Put Playtime First

Typically, before dinner is the best time to get in some playtime. Taking 10 minutes before starting dinner to go out in the yard and play kickball is much better than doing nothing, and you will be surprised at how quickly 10 minutes go by when you are having fun. It will also give you an energy boost after a hard day at work.

When you first start, allow rest breaks during exercise time so that you can accomplish more. Taking small breaks can help you build stamina without getting too tired out. The point is for you and your children to enjoy exercise time!

For children older than six years, exercise time can be once a day. For younger children (two to six years old), try various activities several times a day. Vary the activities and exercises to keep kids challenged. For example, ride your bike on Mondays and Thursdays, walk on Tuesdays, Wednesdays, and Fridays, and play basketball on the weekend.

Get creative about finding a regular time to exercise, and if one person can't make it, don't let that ruin it for everyone else. If the rest of you stay on schedule, the absentee will have an easier time starting up again next time, and everyone will feel better.

▶ HELPFUL HINT: Dress for Success

Choose appropriate clothing and shoes. For most activities, loose clothing and sneakers are fine. If you're just getting started and don't have fancy workout clothes, don't worry about looking or dressing like the professional athletes on TV. The important thing is to get moving. As a reward for your efforts, you may want to buy yourself a new item of workout wear whenever you reach a new exercise goal.

However, if your adolescents or teens are self-conscious about how they look when exercising, make sure they have at least one outfit they can wear to fit in in their exercise "scene," whether it's at the gym or the track.

Important Steps in Exercising

An exercise session should contain several key components: warm-up, stretching, aerobic activity, and cooldown.

Warm-Up

These easy movements slowly increase the blood flow to the working muscles and gradually increase the heart rate. The warm-up prepares the body for the workout.

Stretching

This phase further prepares the muscles for the increased workload and can help with flexibility. Flexibility enables your body to bend, lift, and engage in other activities. Flexibility lessens with age and inactivity. Loss of flexibility reduces the range of motion and interferes with the body's ability to perform daily tasks. Hold all stretches for a slow count of 20, then pause and repeat the stretch.

Get Moving

Appropriate activities for children of all ages are suggested below. Research shows that increasing physical activity levels through daily routines and encouraging regular playtime is most effective for children.

The current recommendation by the American Heart Association is for elementary age children and adolescents to accumulate at least 30 to 60 minutes of age-appropriate activities most days of the week.

Younger age groups (under five years old) focus on intermittent bursts of physical activity for 10 to 15 minutes, alternating moderate to vigorous activity with periods of rest and recovery. This is important for younger individuals because their energy systems are not as well developed as those of adults.

Strength Training

This is most appropriate for adolescents who have reached puberty. Before beginning a strength-training program or working with weights, ask an experienced health professional to help you set up your program. Increasing the strength of the muscles increases the body's ability to burn calories more efficiently and for longer periods of time.

Cooldown

The cooldown is important for the recovery phase. When done properly, it allows the heart to slow down and the muscles to recover. To be certain they've cooled down enough, adults should walk slowly until reaching a heart rate of 20 beats or less in a 10-second time period. Individuals over the age of fifty should have a heart rate of 10 beats or less in a 10-second period before sitting down.

Stretching 101

Why should I stretch?

- Muscles are like rubber bands. They can be stretched only so far before getting sore. If a muscle is stretched beyond what it is able to handle, it can tear. Be careful!

- Stretching allows a muscle to lengthen safely, which helps make your body more flexible.
- Being more flexible allows your body to move better, which means you will perform better at sports and other physical activities.
- Good flexibility helps protect you from getting injured. (Remember the rubber band!)

When should I stretch?

- After warming up, you should stretch before exercising to help your muscles get ready for the activity you are about to do.
- You should also stretch after exercise. Muscles that have been worked will be more flexible and less sore if you stretch after physical activity.

How should I stretch?

- All major muscles that will be used in your activities should be stretched.
- Stretch without moving too much or bouncing. This is called "static" stretching. By holding a stretch, you allow the muscle to lengthen safely.
- Holding a stretch for a slow count of 20 will give you the most benefit. A good stretch may be a little uncomfortable, but it should *never* hurt! If you feel pain, back off a bit until you are not feeling as much discomfort.

When Is Your Child Ready?

Children are always ready to get active—it's never too soon to start. The following list offers a quick overview of age-appropriate activities for various age groups.

- Toddlers: Let them play and run around as much as possible. Short bursts of activity are natural because their bodies are not able to store the large amounts of fuel required to keep going for long periods of time.

At two years of age, a child is typically able to walk on a line, jump, walk up and down stairs, walk on tiptoes, run, stand on one foot, throw a ball overhand, kick a stationary ball, and string large beads.

At three years of age, a child is typically able to hop on one foot, play hop-scotch, ride a push toy, run, turn corners and stop in a simple obstacle course, catch a ball, unbutton buttons, and use scissors.

- Children ages 4 to 6: Keep activities fun. Work on games to promote teamwork and sharing (but don't get bogged down with complicated rules). Key activities at this age promote balance and hand-eye coordination.

At four years of age, a child is typically able to perform a forward roll, gallop, jump over small objects, ride a tricycle or two-wheel bike with training wheels, imitate simple movements, throw a ball underhand, button buttons, and kick a rolling ball.

At five years of age, a child is typically able to skip, ride a bike without training wheels, perform sit-ups and push-ups, jump rope, roller-skate with four wheels, and play T-ball.

- Children ages 6 to 8: Play games with simple rules. Team competitions that promote everyone participating, such as soccer, are important. Team sports provide social interaction and improve self-esteem.
- Children 8 to 12: Play games with more complex rules. Set up activity time with friends. Encourage bike riding around the neighborhood or walking to a friend's house. Team competition helps promote sportsmanship. Promote outdoor activity.
- Children 12 and over: Play tag, backyard football or soccer, and set up regular exercise routines. Team competitions and sports-specific training are popular forms of physical activity. Promote outdoor activity.

Know When Not *to Exercise*

There are times when you should not exercise:

- Avoid exercise when you are sick and have a fever.
- If you or your child has asthma or another chronic illness, check with your doctor regarding an exercise plan prior to starting. If you are sensitive to poor air quality, develop an indoor plan for those days.
- Stop exercising if you experience pain in your chest, dizziness or sickness (nausea or vomiting), cold sweat, or sustained or intense muscle cramps.

Get the Most from Workout Time

Signs of exercising at an appropriate level or intensity include sweating, muscle fatigue, increased heart rate, increased breathing rate, sore muscles the following day, and your rating of how you feel on a perceived exertion scale.

Rating Perceived Exertion (RPE)

10 Very, very Hard
9
8 Very hard
7
6 Hard
5
4 Somewhat hard
3
2 Light
1 Resting

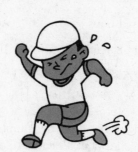

Number 1 on the RPE scale is what you feel like at rest. Moderate intensity is a number 4 to number 6 on the rating scale. Moderate intensity is the goal. If you are just starting an exercise program, then a 2 to 3 on the RPE scale is where you start.

For younger children (two to five years), exercise and activity should cause an increase in breathing, a feeling of being tired, and some sweating.

If you or your children are overweight, another simple way to determine whether you are exercising at an appropriate level is to be able to talk during exercise. If you can't, you may be pushing too hard. Also, you should feel that you are doing a little bit more each time you exercise.

An effective tool for helping track your movement is the pedometer, a simple little device that clips on your waistband and counts the number of steps you take. You may be surprised by how many steps you do—or don't—take every day as part of your regular routine. Kids especially enjoy using these and seeing how their steps add up!

Pedometers are easy to use and can be purchased at sports stores and many general retail stores as well. (Spending a little more for one of better quality will help ensure that it works better and lasts longer.)

To discover how much you are moving and whether you need to increase your activity, wear the pedometer for a couple of days to determine the number of steps you take per day. The following table suggests an average starting point. If you're not there, develop a plan to increase your overall number of steps on a weekly basis.

Workout Ability by Age

AGE RANGE	NUMBER OF STEPS PER DAY
6–12-year-old girls	12,000
6–12-year-old boys	15,000
13–18-year-old girls	At least 10,000
13–18-year-old boys	At least 10,000
Adults (over 18 years of age)	10,000

Source: Study conducted at Arizona State University East, Department of Exercise and Wellness.

If you decide to use walking as a way of working out, try the "step test." Use the pedometer to count the number of steps you can take in 1 minute. The goal is to work out at a rate of at least 3 miles per hour (in other words, a 20-minute mile). (Note: The number of steps may vary slightly depending on your leg length. The package that your pedometer comes in will explain how to adjust your pedometer to match your stride.)

Measure Your Steps

STEPS IN 1 MINUTE	TYPE OF WALK	MINUTES TO WALK 1 MILE
70	2 miles/hour (slow)	30
90	2.5 miles/hour (slow)	24
105	3 miles/hour (moderate)	20
140	4 miles/hour (fast)	15

▶ HELPFUL HINT: Use Your Community Resources

Opportunities to exercise or to participate in physical activity are everywhere. Take advantage of resources such as community centers, Ys, local church or religious institutions, schools, and parks. Your Parks and Recreation Department often provides many outdoor events and other opportunities to get out and get moving.

The Parent's Role

Research at the University of Buffalo by Leonard Epstein and his colleagues showed that when given a choice between physical activity and inactivity (such as watching TV, reading, or playing video games), children who are overweight prefer inactivity. The key to getting kids moving is to provide motivation and rewards for being physically active.

Participating with your child is a very powerful form of motivation. Set a good example: You are never too young or too old to start. Offer praise and encouragement when your child participates in activities with you.

Go for a walk as a family or play Twister or musical chairs. Better yet, plan a family walk after dinner every night—before turning on the TV. (Make TV time a reward only if your family has participated in some sort of physical activity.) If you are watching TV, get up for some physical activity during commercials. For example, you can do simple chores or straightening up. A more fun alternative is to walk around the room until the commercial ends and then sit somewhere new—a modified form of musical chairs. Not only will your children benefit, but you will too. And everyone will enjoy the extra family interaction.

Daily tracking of changes in diet and exercise is important to help everyone see the improvements they have made. It is an excellent motivational tool too. For younger children, a calendar placed on the refrigerator with stickers is a great tracking system. Review the goal calendar often. In fact, some experts recommend reviewing it daily, depending on your family's schedule (perhaps after dinner each night).

Parents play a key role in shaping their children's health habits because children imitate their parents. Take the lead in teaching your child to enjoy staying active and energized.

Setting Your Fitness Goals

Now that you have assessed your and your family's fitness ability, learned about exercise, and identified some new ones to try, it's time to set some goals specific to exercise.

Write one or two goals centered around increasing fitness. Here is an example to get you started:

FAMILY GOALS

	Family	Adults	Child 1	Child 2
Parenting Goal Specific goal: Measure: Time frame:				
Healthy Behaviors Goal Specific goal: Measure: Time frame:				
Healthy Food Goal Specific goal: Measure: Time frame:				
Fitness Goal Specific goal: Measure: Time frame:	We will exercise as a family 2 times, this week			I will ride my bicyle to my friend's house 2 times this week instead of having Mom or Dad drop me off

Go to Appendix A for a full-size copy.

Fiction: I exercise but I don't seem able to lose weight. Why not?

Fact: Weight loss is not the only benefit of exercise. You may be losing inches, have more energy, or sleep better. Be consistent with your exercise program and keep at it. Weight loss will come, especially if you are watching your calorie intake.

PART II

• • •

*Customizing Your Plan for
Your Child's Age Group*

5

• • •

From the Beginning:
Feeding Your Infant

I t is never too early to change your habits, never too early to give your
family a head start, but it is also never too late. This chapter is about the
very beginning, from before conception to your baby's first birthday. The
habits that can lead to obesity can, and often do, develop during your baby's
first year of life. This chapter talks about creating habits that help prevent obesity from developing.

The first years are when food habits and behaviors are developed, and prevention can start even before your baby is conceived. This chapter can serve
as a guide for giving a new baby the best possible start. Answer the following
questions to assess how far along the ROAD to success you are.

Where Are You on the ROAD to Healthy Infant Feeding?

YES   NO   *Check YES or NO to answer the following questions:*

☐ ☐   Did you establish good eating habits for your family prior to your baby being born?

☐ ☐   Have you chosen to breastfeed your infant?

☐ ☐   Would you introduce foods to your child that you are not fond of?

☐ ☐   Do you follow proper portion sizes when feeding your infant?

☐ ☐   Are you feeding your child appropriately according to developmental milestones?

☐ ☐   Have you avoided adding anything to formula or mother's milk in the infant's bottle? (no rice cereal, sugar, baby food, etc.)

☐ ☐   Do you respond to your baby's cues when he or she is full?

☐ ☐   Do you avoid giving your infant sugary drinks or juice?

☐ ☐   Do you plan to use real cups instead of sippy cups?

☐ ☐   Do you avoid propping your baby's bottle?

☐ ☐ Are you avoiding putting a bottle/sippy cup into bed with your baby?

☐ ☐ Do you plan on reintroducing foods to your infant multiple times even if he or she does not like them initially?

_____ *How many yes answers did you have?*

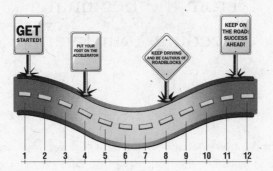

If you scored between 1 and 4, it is time to get your foot on the accelerator and focus on those small changes. If you scored between 5 and 8, you are on the ROAD to better health, but watch out for those roadblocks. If you scored between 9 and 12, use the tips in this chapter to refine and improve your goals or decisions.

Diet and Weight Affect Your Baby's Future

Babies are born knowing how to eat well, so they can naturally grow well. All you have to do is preserve that ability and show them the way. If you help your baby establish a good relationship with food, most of the work toward having a healthy child who grows and eats well will already be done. The importance of having good eating habits is magnified when having a new baby. A healthy lifestyle and healthy weight contribute to:

- having a healthy baby and a healthy pregnancy
- making your children develop good habits (regardless of their genes)
- reducing the risk of obesity in your new family member

Healthy Baby and Mother

The most obvious reason to improve your health before you get pregnant is to have a healthy baby and mother. According to the Surgeon General's Report and the American Academy of Pediatrics (AAP), obesity is associated with negative outcomes. A potential problem is infertility—the inability to have a baby. Furthermore, when the mother is obese during pregnancy, it increases the risks for both mother and the baby. Some of these risks are

- dangerously high blood pressure in the mother
- gestational diabetes (diabetes that develops during pregnancy)
- difficult labor and delivery
- babies that are too big, resulting in the need for a Cesarean section
- low blood sugar in the baby after delivery
- higher chances that the baby will have a neural tube defect like spina bifida

These health risks are absolutely real and make a very compelling reason for mothers to achieve a healthy weight and a healthy lifestyle before trying to conceive. Following the advice from other chapters in this book can help you get on your way to a healthier you, regardless of your age.

If you are already pregnant, however, do not try to lose weight. Weight loss during pregnancy could be dangerous for your baby. All pregnant women need to gain some weight; please talk to your healthcare provider about how much you need to gain. If you are planning to get pregnant in the future, eat well, exercise, and achieve a healthy weight before you start trying to have a baby.

Protecting Your Baby from Obesity

Studies have found that one of the best ways to predict whether a child will be overweight is to look at the mother's weight before becoming pregnant. This means that if the mother is overweight when she gets pregnant, there is an increased probability that her child will grow up to be overweight.

It may be that a mother being obese when the fetus is developing will predispose the child to being overweight. But habits (discussed below in "Being Good Role Models") are extremely important. If your family has poor eating and exercise habits, your baby may be at risk of developing those habits.

The same habits that caused the mother to become overweight are likely to cause overweight in her children. But if your family's habits are healthy, your baby will learn those habits and not have to struggle with the physical, psychological, and emotional consequences of obesity. You have the ability to eliminate the risks that could affect your baby from the very beginning.

Being Good Role Models

Obesity tends to run in families, and genetics do play a role, but obesity is less likely to develop without the behaviors that cause it. Your genes may make your family more likely to be overweight, but you can decrease that risk if you do your part.

Pregnancy is a good incentive to change things for the better. Use this time in your family's life to establish healthy habits. If your family already has good eating and exercise habits by the time the baby comes, you will be giving your baby the best possible start.

Growth During the First Year

One of the first things the doctor will do when assessing your child during checkups is to plot her weight and length on a growth chart. Growth charts are based on established standards for monitoring infant growth. They help you and your healthcare provider follow your child's growth and identify problems that may arise. There are different growth charts for males and females since their growth trends differ.

You should be aware of growth charts and how important they are for monitoring children's growth. Every baby has her own growth curve, which can be tracked from the day she is born by plotting her weight, length, and weight-for-length curves on a growth chart. Babies normally stay on their growth curve as they grow. You can ask your pediatrician to show you your baby's curves, and you can keep track of her growth as part of your baby's medical history. Remember that babies come in all sizes, and that is fine. Do not try to change your child's curves on your own, but do monitor them to make sure she stays on track. If your baby grows consistently and close to her own curves—whatever they are—you can be confident that your child is doing well. If you see a significant jump up or down on any of those curves, then you should discuss this with your primary healthcare provider.

ROAD to Success: Questions for Your Primary Healthcare Provider

- Ask to see growth charts every time you visit.
- Ask what the new plots on the growth curve mean.
- Ask if the curve your child is on is normal and acceptable.

Nutrition and growth are always connected, but feeding will never have more of a role in your child's development—emotional, intellectual, and physical—than during the first year. In order to prevent obesity, it is important to understand the basics of normal infant feeding. Enjoy this exciting time, watch your baby, and follow the cues. Your child will let you know what he or she needs.

Trust your baby to do well. Your child's goal is to grow, master skills, and find his or her place as a member of your family. At this age, your baby's goal is to grow up to be like you, so make sure you are ready to be the best possible role model!

Your Brand-New Baby: 0 to 4 Months

What to Feed Your Baby

According to the American Academy of Pediatrics, the American Dietetic Association, the World Health Organization, and experts all over the world, the best thing you can possibly feed a baby is mother's milk. Nothing else is like it. It is the perfect food for the growth and development of your baby. According to the AAP, infants fed mother's milk may have reduced rates of

- ear infections
- diarrhea
- allergies
- sudden infant death
- diabetes
- lymphoma
- leukemia
- Hodgkin's disease
- asthma
- hypercholesterolemia

Breastfeeding may be a great way to protect your children from becoming overweight. The surgeon general has identified breastfeeding as one of the strategies to decrease the obesity epidemic. More of the benefits of mother's milk are being discovered all the time.

What Is Colostrum?

Colostrum is the highly nutritious liquid that mothers make during the first days after the baby is born. Colostrum is the perfect first food for your baby, providing large amounts of living cells and other immune factors that will defend your baby against many harmful agents. The concentration of these is much higher in colostrum than in mature milk, and infant formula has none.

As the colostrum gradually changes to mature milk during the first weeks after birth, the disease-fighting properties of human milk are still present. In fact, as long as your baby receives your milk, he or she will receive immunological protection against many different viruses and bacteria.

Contraindications for Breastfeeding

Breastfeeding is the optimal feeding method for most babies, but there are a few conditions in which babies should *not* be breastfed. According to the AAP, these conditions are:

- galactosemia in the baby
- active, untreated tuberculosis in the mother
- a human T Cell lymphotropic virus type I or II positive mother
- mothers receiving diagnostic or therapeutic radioactive isotopes
- mothers exposed to radioactive materials
- mothers taking certain medications until the medication has cleared the milk
- mothers abusing drugs
- mothers with active herpes simplex lesions on the breast
- HIV infection in the mother

When breastfeeding is not possible, infant formula is the only alternative. No other milk is acceptable, including goat's milk, whole milk, or evaporated milk. Babies fed infant formula tend to be bigger and consume more calories than babies fed mother's milk. Your baby can grow well on formula alone for the first four to six months of life, but there are some special things you need to do to protect your baby from overfeeding when you use a bottle. These will be discussed later in this chapter.

How Often to Feed Your Baby

Feed your baby often, especially in the very beginning. New babies need to eat eight to twelve times per day to meet their needs, whether they are breast-fed or formula-fed. If you have a sleepy or very contented baby, he may not wake up for feedings. If your newborn is sleeping for more than 4 hours at a stretch, you will need to wake him.

Some new mothers are afraid they will not be able to make enough milk, or feel unsure about whether they are "doing it right." But the baby will let you know when and how much he needs to eat. Feed your baby on demand day and night and your milk will become sufficient. The vast majority of women are capable of producing all the milk their babies need. Follow your baby's cues to eat, and remember that breastfeeding discomfort should be minimal. You are doing it right if your baby is growing and you are free from pain. However, if you have any concerns, ask to see a lactation consultant, who is a breastfeeding expert and who can be a wonderful source of help and support.

You'll probably find that once you and your baby get past the first few days, you'll be well on your way to a successful breastfeeding experience.

Breastfeeding Tips: For the Journey Ahead

- **Breastfeeding should begin within the first hour after delivery.** Breastfeeding should begin as early as the first hour after delivery. If you are unable to start breastfeeding right away, pumping can be an option. The early days of lactation are critical, but with good support, breastfeeding can still be initiated for several weeks after delivery.
- **A proper latch-on is crucial for success.** Good latch-on will help ensure proper emptying and milk supply. If latch-on is not correct it can cause problems down the road.
- **Newborns should remain with the mother.** It is not necessary to separate healthy babies from their mothers. Having the baby close by will facilitate timely breastfeeding and ease in establishing milk supply.
- **Babies should be positioned for comfort.** Assuring that your baby is positioned properly will help both your comfort and hers throughout the feeding. Positioning the baby so that her head requires minimal turning will help ease the suck and swallow reflexes. Positioning also means that you are comfortable with proper support from pillows.
- **Avoid artificial nipples.** During the first weeks when your milk supply is starting to be established, avoid artificial nipples. This will help establish the milk supply, as the baby will work hard to help get the milk let down. Babies may also become frustrated when they are given a fast-flowing artificial nipple and then placed back on the breast at another feeding.
- **Feed the baby frequently.** Initially your baby may want to be fed every 1½ to 2½ hours. During the first month, a baby who sleeps more than 4 hours during the day or night should probably be awakened to feed. After the first month, a baby who is gaining weight should be allowed to sleep and eat on demand.
- **Feed from both breasts.** It is recommended to offer milk from both breasts. Allow the baby to feed on one breast until he or she finishes or pulls away, and then offer the other breast. Most but not all babies will feed from both breasts during each feeding. You should alternate the breast you start with at each feeding.

Know Where to Go for Help

Learn as much as you can about breastfeeding. You don't have to have all the answers, but you should definitely know where to go if you need help.

1. Find a friend, neighbor, or coworker who has breastfed successfully. She can offer you tips for success and support.
2. If you feel you need professional help or would like to see a lactation consultant, check with your hospital. The hospital should have consultants available to you, or try this Web site—www.ilca.org—to find a certified lactation consultant. Your local WIC (Women, Infants, and Children) office, the La Leche League (www.lalecheleague.org), and www.breastfeeding.org are also good sources of help.
3. You can find a local support group at the La Leche League that can help you get through this and may even help you find breastfeeding-friendly daycare. Your hospital should have the number, but you can call 1-800-LALECHE or go to their Web site.
4. Find a good-quality breast pump (if you need one).

Breastfeeding for the Working Mother

Many mothers think that they cannot breastfeed because they have to return to work. Remember that you are truly working for only part of the day, but you are still very much a full-time mom twenty-four hours a day. Pump when away from your baby and breastfeed your baby when you come home. You and your baby don't have to sacrifice breastfeeding because of employment. You *can* make it work!

Here are some perceived roadblocks and how to overcome them:

- **If I breastfeed, it will be hard for the baby once I go back to work.** Babies are very resilient. You can definitely breastfeed your baby before and after returning to work. If you wait to introduce a bottle until your breastfeeding is well established (usually around three weeks after birth), your baby should switch back and forth from breast to bottle.
- **My job is not favorable toward supportive breastfeeding.** Talk to your employer as early as possible and try to work out an arrangement. It always helps if you have a plan for making things work for both of you. You may have already seen a room you can use for pumping and figured out what times are the most convenient for you to take your breaks. You can pump during your lunch, or you can

explain that while other employees take smoking breaks, you will be taking pumping breaks (these may be longer than smoking breaks, but you don't need as many, and it won't cost the company anything).

• **What if my baby is in childcare?** All childcare situations should be supportive of parental feeding choices, but not all of them are. Do some research, ask questions, and find a center close to your home or work that you know will respect your choice. There is no reason to treat a breastfed baby any differently from a bottle-fed one. The milk does not need a special refrigerator or special precautions. Each baby needs to get his or her own specified feedings, whether they consist of breastmilk or a specific kind of formula.

Does my baby need anything else? Talk to your pediatrician about the need to give your baby a vitamin or mineral supplement. Other than the vitamins or minerals that your healthcare provider may recommend, your baby needs nothing else at this age. Your baby does not need cereal, syrup, yogurt, any other foods, or water. Mother's milk and properly mixed formula have enough water to meet your child's needs. Your baby does not need juice!

Introducing solids too early, before 4 to 6 months, is not a good idea. It can result in constipation, allergies, poor growth, overweight, and missing out on important nutrients in breastmilk or formula. Babies that young are not ready, developmentally, for solid food. They probably can't eat from a spoon yet, and it is never a good idea to add food to your baby's bottle.

How to Feed Your Baby

Your newborn is very wise and knows how much and how often he needs to eat to grow well. The only thing babies can't do is tell you with words, but they do communicate with you all the time. Watch your baby. He gives you clues about his needs. Every baby has a different temperament and different way of communicating. Observing your baby closely will help you get to know his signals. Here are some signs babies may give when they are getting hungry:

• sucking on their hands or blanket
• moving or licking their lips
• turning their head toward your hand when touched on the cheek
• may be more awake or active
• may simply have an interested facial expression.

You cannot spoil your newborn by responding to his needs. Young babies cannot manipulate you. They are simply telling you what they need. Responding to their needs lets them know they will be taken care of and builds their trust.

Fussing and crying are usually signs that something is wrong. Some babies fuss or cry to signal that they are hungry without giving other noticeable clues, but for most babies, crying is a late sign of hunger. If you feel that the earliest clue your baby gives you is crying, his early cues may just be extrasubtle. Look again, watch for a change in his state or "mood." He may just stare at you intently or be very interested in your face, and may even give cues when still asleep.

Many books suggest that babies should have a schedule—even at this age—and it is understandable why having one is comforting for parents. But the truth is that your baby should be in charge of his schedule for now. You will find that your baby gradually settles into a schedule that you can predict. As your baby gets older, you will start having more control and will start to develop your role as a parent in regard to nutrition.

Hunger Spurts or Growth Spurts

The La Leche League advises, "There will be times when your baby will want to eat more often. It doesn't mean that your milk supply is low. He may just be going through one of these spurts. You can expect these to occur at about 3 weeks, 6 weeks, 3 months and 6 months old, but your baby may be somewhat different. The most important thing is not to panic, just ride it out, and continue to breastfeed on demand. Growth spurts usually last only 2–3 days, and feeding on demand helps you keep up with your baby's growing needs. Resist the urge to give him or her a bottle. This will not help the two of you to stay 'in sync.' Remember, if your baby is growing well, you are making enough milk."

How Do You Know If Your Baby Is Getting Enough to Eat?

Ask yourself this one question: Is my baby growing well? If the answer is yes, you don't need to be concerned about how much she is getting. If your new baby is producing about six wet diapers and several stools per day, she is probably getting enough. But growth is the best measure: If your baby is growing well and following her growth curves, she is getting enough, and that is all that matters.

Another concern is fullness. Babies give clear signs that they are full. They stop sucking, spit out the nipple, or fall asleep. They indicate to you when they are done eating, so your job is not to overfeed.

It is less likely for the breastfed baby to be overfed. These babies have full control because mothers cannot urge them to finish every last drop. This may be a reason why breastfeeding protects your baby from being overweight.

Bottle-feeding, on the other hand, allows overfeeding because the caretaker—not the baby—is in control of the feeding. Another way that babies eat more than they want or need is if you add foods, like rice cereal or syrup, to their bottles, whether it contains formula or mother's milk. Not following the formula's preparation instructions is another way to overfeed babies. Always follow the manufacturer's instruction. These instructions may change, so make sure you read them carefully.

Fortunately, extra calories can be avoided by offering mother's milk alone or formula prepared following the manufacturer's instructions. Removing the bottle when your baby "tells" you that he or she is full is the key during these early months to prevent your baby being overweight down the road.

▶ HELPFUL HINT: Avoid the "Clean Plate" Club
Resist the urge to get your baby to finish that last bit left in the bottle, even if the bottle contains precious breastmilk. This will cause him to be less sensitive to the natural cues of fullness that cause him to stop feeding on his own.

Interacting with your baby during feeding is crucial to establish a good feeding relationship. Your baby needs your attention. Whether he is breastfed or bottle-fed, he needs you to be engaged. Hold your baby during feedings. Be sure to look at, and stroke your baby, and watch his movements. Enjoy feeding your baby. You will quickly notice that he craves this attention from you. Propping up a bottle robs you both of this experience, can result in overfeeding, and can lead to choking.

Bottle-Feeding Guidelines

If your baby is taking a bottle (with mother's milk or formula), keep these important tips in mind:

- The only thing that should ever be given in a bottle is mother's milk or infant formula. Do not offer anything else in a bottle—not water or juice.
- Do not alter the milk's composition in any way by adding cereal, syrup, or sugar. Nothing should be added to mother's milk, and formula should be prepared according to the manufacturer's instructions.

There may be some exceptions to these guidelines. If your baby has a special need, your healthcare provider may suggest that you add something to the bottle. But those cases are rare and your healthcare provider would be the one to tell you what to do—never add food or alter mixing instructions on your own.

Introducing Solids: 4 to 6 Months

When Is the Best Time to Start Giving Your Baby Solid Food?

The American Academy of Pediatrics and the American Dietetic Association recommend that you wait until about six months of age to introduce any other foods. This maximizes the benefits your baby receives from breastmilk, because he or she will drink more. Introducing solids may decrease the amount of breastmilk your baby wants to drink, so he or she may miss some of those precious benefits.

If your baby is formula-fed, you can start experimenting with solids between 4 and 6 months of age. Determine the exact timing by your baby's readiness. Babies typically show readiness for solids when they

- can sit with some support
- can grab things and put them in their mouth
- can turn their head away to tell you they have had enough
- do not push the spoon or food out with the tongue
- can make chewing movements by moving the mouth up and down

If your baby does not yet show these signs, wait for her to be ready. There is no need to rush. At this age, most of her nutrition should still come from breastmilk or formula. Do not give in to peer pressure and start your baby on solids too early. Every mother is told that some other baby "accomplished" something earlier. Starting solids too early is nothing to be proud of. However, you can definitely be proud of following your baby's cues and signs for readiness.

> *Margie wanted to add rice cereal to her baby's bottle-feeding, as her friend told her it made her child sleep through the night. Margie's doctor advised her against this practice. He told Margie that her two-month-old baby was too young to have anything other than mother's milk or formula. Margie stopped adding rice cereal and two weeks later her son started to sleep more hours in the night all on his own.*

What to Feed Your Baby and How Much

By the age of six months, babies need a source of iron in their diet. Baby rice cereal is the most common first food, because it is unlikely to cause allergies and is fortified with iron. Start with baby rice cereal, and once he has had rice cereal for about a week without any signs of allergies, you can offer another kind of baby cereal, like oat or barley. Offer baby cereal twice a day and only after you have recently finished breastfeeding or bottle-feeding.

Be patient and respect your baby's likes and dislikes by not pushing him to eat something he doesn't want at that time. However, do offer it again, and again, and again at different meals and different days. It may take several tries for him to like a particular food, sometimes as many as ten to fifteen tries. That is normal, and your job is to keep *presenting* your baby with foods.

If your baby likes the food, offer him as much as he wants. Babies between four and six months usually eat only 1 to 2 tablespoons of cereal per day. If you wait until your baby is ready to eat solids, he will be able to let you know when he has had enough, by refusing to open his mouth, turning away, spitting food out, or crying—in case you missed earlier cues.

Your baby needs all the nutrition he or she can get from mother's milk or formula, and breastmilk and formula have enough water to satisfy thirst. Giving water or juice can decrease a baby's intake of breastmilk or formula and cause poor growth. Your baby will still need breastmilk or formula every time solids are offered—offer milk or formula before solids. Your baby should also drink breastmilk or formula at other times to satisfy thirst and other needs.

Don't add salt, sugar, syrup, or honey to your baby's food. The food may taste bland to you, but when your baby is just learning about food, he or she needs to know food's natural flavors. Salt, sugar, and other seasonings also add extra sodium and carbohydrates that your baby does not need. They may even cause some harm by causing diarrhea, or exposing your baby to dangerous bacteria or toxins.

▶ ROADBLOCK: Honey—Not for Infants

You may think that honey is a "natural" food and therefore safe to add to infant formula or food to enhance the flavor or add calories. But honey should not be consumed by infants less than two years of age. Honey contains toxic spores of *Clostridium botulinum* that infants' gastrointestinal tracts are not developed enough to fight off.

SERVING SIZES FOR YOUR INFANT

	Birth to 4 Months	4–6 Months	6–8 Months	8–10 Months	10–12 Months
Expressed breastmilk* or infant formula	8–12 feedings 2–6 ounces per feeding (18–32 ounces per day)	4–6 feedings 4–6 ounces per feeding (27–45 ounces per day)	3–5 feedings 6–8 ounces per feeding (24–32 ounces per day)	3–4 feedings 7–8 ounces per feeding (24–32 ounces per day)	24–32 ounces of breastmilk or formula per day
Cereal, bread, and starches	None	2–3 servings of iron-fortified baby rice cereal mixed with breastmilk or formula (do not mix with juice) (serving=1–2 tbsp)	2–3 servings of iron-fortified baby cereal and other soft, cooked breads, cereals, and starches (serving=1–2 tbsp)	2–3 servings of iron-fortified baby cereal and other soft, cooked breads, cereals, and starches (serving=1–2 tbsp)	4 servings breads and other soft starches; iron-fortified baby cereal (serving =1–2 tbsp)
Fruits and vegetables	None	None	Begin to offer plain cooked, mashed, or strained baby food vegetables and fruits. Avoid combination meat and vegetable dinners	2–3 servings of soft, cut up, and mashed vegetables and fruits daily (serving=1–2 tbsp)	4 servings daily of fruits and vegetables (serving=2–3 tbsp)
Meats and other protein foods	None	None	None	Begin to offer well-cooked, soft, finely cut or pureed meats, cheese, and casseroles	1–2 ounces daily of soft, finely cut or chopped meat or other protein foods

*If your baby is breastfeeding, his or her pattern may be different from that of a bottle-fed baby. That is okay. There is no need to restrict the number of times you breastfeed your baby.

Your baby will let you know when he or she has had enough. This may be after the first bite, or even after just looking at the food on the spoon. He or she may want to eat a lot. Let your baby have control. The serving sizes table has information about how much a baby usually eats, but it is just a rough guide. Most babies eat very little one time and more at other times; yours may love cereal or may not. Respect your baby's choices!

Is Your Baby's Tummy Empty or Full?

Babies typically start out hungry, and as they get full, they gradually start losing interest in their food. These are some signs you can look for to avoid overfeeding:

HUNGRY BABY	BABY HAS HAD ENOUGH
Very interested in food	Interested in things other than food
Opens mouth to receive food	Closes mouth when food approaches
Body leans toward food	Moves away from spoon or bottle
Excited about food approaching mouth	Swats food away, spits food out
Crying (for food)	Crying (to stop the feeding)

How Should the Baby Be Fed?

Mother's milk or formula are the only things that should go in a bottle. All solid food should be given in a spoon. If your baby is exclusively breastfed, she may never use a bottle in her life—that's good because you will never have to deal with getting your baby to stop drinking from a bottle.

If your baby has been drinking from a bottle that contains only mother's milk or formula, you actually help her when it comes time to develop the skills to drink from a cup. Learning to drink properly from a real cup is a developmental milestone that is often underestimated. Transitioning your baby at an appropriate age will protect her teeth and avoid the extremely difficult task of getting a 14-, 16-, 24-, or even a 36-month-old child to stop drinking from a bottle or sippy cup.

Moving Along: 6 to 8 Months

Now your baby is six months old and probably ready for solids. He or she should show you all the signs for readiness that were discussed in the previous stage and maybe even more. He or she may even start to be interested in what you are eating!

You should start from the beginning, though, with rice cereal. Introduce any new food for about a week to watch for allergies, then offer another food, and repeat the same precaution every time you give a new food. At six to eight months of age, your baby can have other foods, and now your baby needs iron. Babies are born with iron stores that last for about six months. Unfortified cereal, fruits, and vegetables are not good sources of iron, so cereal that is fortified with iron is a good source to meet their needs.

Check the serving sizes table for some guidelines on how much he or she might need. If your baby is refusing baby cereals or not eating enough of them, do not be pushy. You can check with your pediatrician, who may recommend some iron drops.

If your baby was not fed breastmilk, he may or may not have eaten cereals; it depends on whether he was ready for them or not (check the list of signs of readiness earlier in this chapter). Your baby probably wants to feed himself now. Here is what to look for to make sure your baby is ready for this change:

- Can sit without support.
- Can grab things with hands and put them in his mouth.
- Can hold a bottle.
- Can drink from a cup! (It may be messy and your baby may need a little help, but as long as he can do it, you should let him.)

What to Feed Your 6- to 8-Month Old

At this age, babies can be introduced to a whole new world of foods—fruits, vegetables, breads, crackers, and cereal. Remember to offer a new food for about a week before you try another new food. However, once a food is "safe," meaning no allergies show up, it can be offered with another "safe" food from your baby's ever-growing repertoire of safe foods. If your baby dislikes a food, don't push him or her, but do continue to offer it over and over again.

You don't need to buy commercial baby food; you can prepare your own if you want. Fruits and vegetables should be cooked and then pureed. Start with very smooth purees and gradually progress to coarser and coarser textures depending on what your baby can swallow as he or she grows.

At this age your baby can technically have other liquids in addition to formula; however, it is not necessary to give anything other than breastmilk or formula. Your child is perfectly capable of eating fruits and vegetables; he or she doesn't need to drink calories from sugar (natural or added) in juice or other beverages. However, if you give juice to your baby occasionally, limit the amount to a maximum of 4 ounces per day and offer it in a real cup, not a sippy cup.

Of course, soda and juice drinks are a no-no. Sugary drinks, including juice, are one of the biggest contributors to excess calorie consumption leading to obesity. It is easiest to spare children the trouble by never getting them started on juice: they just don't need that in their diet.

How Much to Feed

You are already well on your way to establishing your role as a parent. Your baby has a predictable need for breastfeeding or drinking formula, and you are feeding solids twice a day. Now it's time to increase the frequency. You are in charge of the schedule for solids. Feed your baby solids three to five times a day (remember to include breastfeeding or formula with the "meals"), whatever times work best for your schedule.

You are responsible for choosing what types of foods you offer (including breastmilk or formula). The baby is in charge of deciding whether to eat or not, and how much.

Look at the serving sizes table on page 106 for some ideas on what foods to offer, but don't be pushy with any kind of food. If you offer a balanced menu and are not pushy or nervous about any foods, your child will chose a balanced diet.

When parents push one food and limit another, children start wanting more of the restricted food and less of the food you are pushing them to eat. You may think you are being very subtle or sneaky, but children are smart and will figure it out. Trust your baby to eat well.

How to Feed

This is a very fun stage. Your baby will start trying to feed herself! She can grab a cracker or piece of toast to munch on it until it is soft enough to swallow. Watch carefully to make sure she doesn't bite off more than she can safely handle. If your baby shows signs that she wants to feed herself, let her. You can put small pieces of food (even pureed food or very small pieces of soft-cooked veggies) on the tray of the high chair and let her pick them up and put them in her mouth while you continue to feed with a spoon. This can be adorable to watch, but it probably won't be clean! Enjoy your growing baby—that pleasure will make up for some of the mess.

Once a baby wants to feed herself, you can still try to feed her yourself, but take her cues. If you fight your baby's attempts, she may not eat as well or may stop trying to feed herself altogether. Neither is desirable. Encourage a little independent spirit.

During this age your baby will reach two very important milestones: being able to hold a bottle and drink from a cup. Your baby's ability to hold her own bottle is great and is okay to do during feedings. Only one temptation must be resisted, and it's one that someone will eventually suggest as a wonderful idea: Do not leave a bottle (or two or three) in your baby's crib for her to grab and eat during the night.

Your desire for the baby to sleep through the night is strong. But if your baby is waking up during the night because she is truly hungry, a parent should be there to feed her and make sure she is safe. If she isn't hungry, but eats for comfort, it can cause a lot more harm than good. A bottle in the crib can cause tooth decay, poor food intake, and poor growth, and can lead to obesity.

The ability to drink from a cup is often underutilized. Babies can be messy when they eat, but they need the practice to get better. Your baby can certainly try to drink breastmilk or formula from a real cup. Skip the sippy cups;

they are just a bottle in disguise. (Read Chapter 6 for more in-depth information about sippy cups.)

Your Older Baby: 8 to 12 Months

By now, your baby is on the way to becoming a child who eats well enough to grow well. Ideally you have helped him or her develop the healthy habits discussed to this point. But if something is wrong, rest assured that children are very resilient and want to do well at everything. It's never too late to introduce them to good habits for healthy eating.

When to Feed

Your baby is ready to move on to the next stage of feeding when he:

- can chew by moving his mouth in circles (close to the way an adult chews)
- tries to feed himself and grab the spoon from you
- can lick food from his lower lip

What to Feed

Your baby can probably eat a large variety of cereals, fruits, and vegetables. Now you can add beans, meats, yogurt, and cheese to her diet. Just as before, add one food a week to make sure she has no allergic reactions. Then keep adding a new food each week.

You are also a pro at letting your baby decide how much to eat of any food at any given meal. Ideally, by now you have figured out a fairly regular schedule for solids: about four times a day is usually adequate. Breastmilk and formula should still be offered on demand, but solid food should naturally and gradually increase in quantity.

How to Feed

Now the final piece of the puzzle, how to feed your child. The time has come to bring your baby to the family table. If he was eating with your family at the table earlier, well done. But if not, now is the time to let him be part of the family. He will show you how much he wants to do this with some signs. You may see him:

- reaching for your plate
- wanting to drink from your glass

- not wanting to be fed anymore
- refusing his food if it is different from yours

Your child will gradually be able to eat everything you eat. He can eat pasta, vegetables, meat, cookies, crackers, yogurt, cheese, breakfast cereal, pancakes, fruit, and much more. His menu can start to look the same as yours, assuming that your menu at home is balanced. You must give your young one small pieces of soft foods that he can safely handle on his own, but you can still feed him while he works on feeding himself—if your baby lets you.

Breastfeeding is still the best nutrition you can give your baby. Breastmilk continues to benefit your child for as long as you and your baby decide to continue to breastfeed. The American Academy of Pediatrics and every major health organization strongly recommend that all babies receive their mother's milk for *at least* a year, and after a year, for as long as you like.

Your child also can start drinking breastmilk or formula from a cup, which can ease him into the next big change—no more bottles. By the age of one, your baby should stop drinking infant formula and stop using a bottle. You can introduce whole milk in a cup (not a bottle). If the only drink he has ever had in a bottle is formula, he will associate whole milk with his cup, which will make eliminating formula and bottles much easier. You can—and should—say "bye-bye, bottle" by the age of one. There is no age at which your baby should stop breastfeeding or drinking breastmilk, but he should still stop using a bottle by the first birthday.

It is important that your baby reach the milestones of drinking from a cup and not using a bottle now. The longer bottle drinking goes on, the harder it is to stop.

▶ ROADBLOCK: What to Do if Your Child Cries or Throws a Fit
The same thing you would do if she were throwing a fit to get you to give her a kitchen knife: Do not give in. Bottles are obviously not dangerous, but you would never let your child manipulate you into doing something that might harm her, and that is the point. If the fits do not ever work, your child will quickly learn they are not worth the effort, and the fits will stop. Help your child do well!

Your baby wants to grow up at this age. If you wait too long, he or she may not be as interested in reaching this milestone, and it can become a greater struggle.

After your baby's first birthday, he or she is not longer an infant. This chapter helped you establish a solid base for a lifetime of healthy habits. And if you follow your child's lead, you will gradually transition the eating and feeding relationship from one of dependence to one of independence for your child.

The future may have some new challenges for you, but a healthy lifestyle is much easier to maintain if you have mastered the basics. The next chapters show you how to continue helping your child maintain a healthy relationship with food, have positive meal interactions, and gradually learn to take care of himself or herself. Enjoy the ride!

Setting Your Infant Feeding Goals

Now create your personalized goals on the Family Goals table in Appendix A. These may be actions you'll take to help yourself and your own health, as well as what you can do to help your baby.

Sample goals for you and your baby:

- I will retry a food this week that my child did not previously like.
- I will not give my eight-month-old more than 4 ounces of juice per day.
- I will make a conscious effort to observe and act upon my baby's feeding cues every day.

Fiction: My child needs more food. He cries all the time for food, so I give him Cheerios or Goldfish.

Fact: Parents sometimes misinterpret their child's cues. A child may cry or complain due to boredom, anger, wanting attention, or something else. Most of the reasons for crying, especially in toddlers, do not relate to food. Yet parents may use food as a way to keep their child quiet.

Children need no more than three meals a day and two scheduled snacks (planned in advance). By allowing your child to "graze" on finger foods through-out the day, you are increasing caloric intake beyond what's needed. The human body is not designed to graze all day in the way that cattle are.

6

• • •

Setting Good Habits with
the Pre-K Set

As toddlers start to take on their own personalities, they also start to develop their own opinions about foods. The key is that you are providing a well-balanced diet from a variety of foods and continue to offer healthy foods that they may not have liked on previous attempts. Answer the following questions to assess how far along the ROAD to success you are in providing nutritious intake for your toddler.

Where Are You on the ROAD to Raising a Healthy Toddler and Preschooler?

YES NO *Check YES or NO to answer the following questions:*

☐ ☐ Is your child drinking all beverages from a cup?

☐ ☐ If your child is two or older, have you transitioned from whole to 2% milk?

☐ ☐ Are you aware of proper portion sizes for your child's age?

☐ ☐ Do you let your child eat independently?

☐ ☐ Do you continue to offer foods that your child previously disliked?

☐ ☐ Do you avoid making your child clean the plate?

☐ ☐ Do you involve your child in making healthy choices while grocery shopping?

☐ ☐ Do you limit your child to no more than 4–6 ounces of juice per day?

☐ ☐ Do you make certain that your child is offered a variety of foods?

☐ ☐ Are you aware of the meals and snacks that are offered at your childcare center?

☐ ☐ Do you have set meal- and snacktimes?

☐ ☐ Do you offer nonfood rewards to your child (trips to the park, stickers, etc.)?

_____ *How many yes answers did you have?*

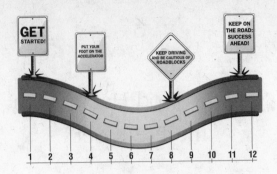

If you scored between 1 and 4, it is time to get your foot on the accelerator and focus on making small changes. If you scored between 5 and 8, you are on the ROAD to better health, but be careful of those roadblocks. If you scored between 9 and 12, use the tips in this chapter to refine and improve your goals or decisions.

Healthy Growth and Development
Growth and Physical Development

By the first birthday, children have usually doubled their birth weight. By two years of age, their weight on average is four times their birth weight. After the age of two, children's growth begins to slow down, and their appetite decreases. The amount of food they eat can be unpredictable. Remember to be aware of hunger and fullness cues that your child displays at this age. It is normal if the amount of food your child consumes decreases. Between the ages of two and five years, children gain an average of 4½ to 6½ pounds a year and grow 2½ to 3½ inches per year.

Nutrition and Feeding Skill Development

Each child is an individual and develops at a different pace. Keep that in mind when looking at the tables on pages 115 and 117–118. These are intended as rough guides, not rules about where your child should be. As the Feeding Skills Development table outlines, by age one, children should begin weaning from the bottle and drinking from a cup. This is the age when they are able to move their tongue from side to side to move food in order to chew it better. By age one, children also can begin finger feeding using their thumb and index finger, called a "pincer grasp."

Between twelve and fifteen months of age, children should transition from infant formula to regular whole milk. At fifteen months of age, children usually can drink from a cup using one or both hands. Youngsters this age

FEEDING SKILLS DEVELOPMENT

Feeding Skill Development	Years 1	2	3	4	5	Food Advancement to Meet Feeding Skills
Transitions from bottle to cup Holds cup and drinks with help, some spillage Reaches for spoon Bites and chews with coordination Uses pincer grasp (thumb and index finger) Uses fingers to scrape food toward self Grasps food with hands (self-feeds)	▓					Formula to whole milk or toddler formula Increase protein foods (e.g., whole egg, yogurt, cheese) Stage 3 baby foods to soft, mashed, or ground table/finger foods (e.g., mashed potatoes, macaroni and cheese, puddings, crackers)
Holds spoon palm down Scoops food with spoon with spillage Brings spoon to mouth with spillage May start using small fork Holds cup handle and drinks without lid Ability to chew varies with firmness and texture of foods Unwraps foods		▓				Whole milk or 2% milk Decreased milk intake (will provide less than ½ of daily nutrients) Soft pieces of food to prick with a fork (stew, noodles, vegetables, small chopped pieces of meat)
Drinks from open cup without spillage Combines eating with fingers and utensils Pours liquids from small containers			▓			Raisins, hot dogs, peanut butter, and other foods no longer choking hazard Use small plastic pitcher and cup for pouring
Feeds self well using spoon and fork Eats a variety of foods and textures Drinks while holding straw Helps with food preparation (vegetables) Sets utensils on table for eating Serves food on plate using spoon				▓		Serving sizes will increase Spread butter or peanut butter on bread Raw fruits Able to dip fruits and vegetables Salad (tear lettuce and grate carrots) Layer foods to make sandwich (e.g., cheese and crackers) Open cereal box Assist with snacks
Independent self-feeder with fork Serves food and passes for sharing Chews with lips closed Cuts with knife Opens food containers and removes food					▓	Eating a variety of foods from each of the food groups with mixed textures Ongoing process introducing child to new foods and textures

also begin using a spoon. Notice that your child wants to feed himself or herself as much as possible. By eighteen months, your child should be able to use a spoon with foods that can stick to the spoon, such as yogurt, mashed potatoes, cooked cereals, and puddings. Avoid allowing your child to walk around with a sippy cup. Although the sippy cup is convenient and less of a mess, it can be a source of extra calories. If you do choose to use one, fill it with plain water.

By two years of age, toddlers begin drinking from an open cup without dribbling. They can bite, chew, and grind food. Children this age also have developed the skill to swallow foods of different textures. This is the time when you may allow your child to begin using a fork. After the age of three, youngsters may begin eating foods such as raisins and peanut butter, but only if you feel that your child will not choke on them. By three or four years of age, toddlers are usually able to combine finger feeding and have become more proficient with the use of a spoon or fork.

Beware Potential Choking Hazards

These foods are considered choking hazards and should not be offered until after the age of three:

- peanut butter
- hot dogs
- popcorn
- nuts
- raisins
- whole grapes
- hard candy
- raw carrots
- marshmallows
- ice cubes
- gum

At four years of age, children should be able to serve and feed themselves well, with little spilling. They also should be able to pour liquids from a container into a cup. By five, children should be independent feeders and probably have mastered all of these skills. They are also old enough to be able to set the table and other meal-related activities. It is a great time to start fostering interest and involvement with meals.

Understanding Foods and Portions for Children

Understanding serving portion sizes along with making good food choices is a part of healthy eating. First, know how much food your child is eating, as extra calories may lead to excessive weight gain. Then focus on good choices in each of the food groups, increasing variety as your toddler grows.

TODDLERS TO EARLY SCHOOL AGE

Food Groups and Number of Daily Servings	Age 12–23 Months*	Age 2–3 Years*	Age 4–6 Years	Age 7–8 Years
Milk and Milk Products *Low-fat or fat-free milk or milk products*	2 cups/day (whole milk or milk products)	2 cups/day (whole milk or milk products)	2–3 cups/day	2–3 cups/day
	1 cup = 1 cup of milk or yogurt, 1½ ounces of neutral cheese, 2 ounces of processed cheese, ⅓ cup of shredded cheese			
Meat and Other Protein Foods *Includes beef, chicken, pork, poultry, fish, eggs, peanut butter, and legumes*	1½ ounces/day	2–4 ounces/day	3–5 ounces/day	4–5 ounces/day
	1 ounce of meat = 1 ounce of beef, poultry or fish, ¼ cup cooked beans 1 egg, 1 tablespoon peanut butter,† ½ ounce of nuts†			
Breads, Cereals, and Starches *Includes whole-grain breads, infant and cooked cereals, rice, pasta, ready-to-eat cereals. Half of all starches should be whole grains*	2 ounces/day	3–5 ounces/day	4–5 ounces/day	4–5 ounces/day
	1 ounce = 1 slice whole-grain bread, ½ cup cooked cereal, rice or pasta, 1 cup dry cereal			
Fruits *Includes one source of vitamin C daily (citrus fruits and juices, strawberries) and one source of vitamin A every other day (dark green and yellow fruits, melons)*	1 cup/day	1–1½ cup/day	1–1½ cup/day	1½ cup/day
	1 cup = 1 cup of fruit or 100% fruit juice, ½ cup of dried fruit (limit juice to 4–6 ounces of juice/day)			
Vegetables *Includes one source of vitamin C daily (broccoli, tomatoes, and potatoes) and one source of vitamin A every other day (spinach, sweet potatoes, corn, squash)*	¾ cup/day	1–1½ cup/day	1½–2 cups/day	1½–2½ cups/day
	1 cup = 1 cup of raw or cooked vegetables or vegetable juice, 2 cups of raw leafy greens			

(continued)

TODDLERS TO EARLY SCHOOL AGE (*continued*)

Food Groups and Number of Daily Servings	Age 12–23 Months*	Age 2–3 Years*	Age 4–6 Years	Age 7–8 Years
Fats and Oils *Includes margarine, butter, oils*	Do not limit	3 servings/day	4–5 servings/day	4–5 servings/day
	1 serving = 1 teaspoon oil, margarine, butter, or mayonnaise 1 tablespoon salad dressing, sour cream, or light mayonnaise			
Miscellaneous *Desserts, sweets, soft drinks, candy, jams, and jelly.*	**Limit to small amount, use sparingly**			

Source: Created by Texas Children's Hospital, adapted by the United States Department of Agriculture.
NOTE: One serving is equivalent to the quantity listed in each age appropriate box
*For younger children, the portions will be smaller but amounts are for total intake per day (i.e., 3 – ¼ cup servings of vegetables = ¾ cup for day).
†Not recommended for children under 3 years of age.

Milk and Milk Products

By twelve months of age, children should transition from formula to whole milk. They also may begin eating other dairy products like yogurt and cheese. By two, children should begin transitioning to low-fat milk products. Before the age of two, children need extra fat to promote appropriate growth and brain development. If your child is already exhibiting signs of obesity, chances are he is getting enough fat from other sources and your primary care provider may recommend reducing milk at an earlier age or possibly switching to skim or fat free.

By two years of age, most children no longer need extra fat. Making the switch at an early age is much easier than doing it when your child is older and more likely to notice and be resistant to switching to low-fat milk. Still, even with a younger child, you can make a gradual switch, going first to 2% milk and then later to 1% milk or skim milk.

An early switch to low-fat milk also helps promotes these habits for a long time. Your child will be more likely to continue to drink low-fat milk as a teen and adult, instead of higher fat and calorie whole milk.

However, if your child is underweight and is not getting enough calories and fat from other foods, then he may need to remain on whole milk if advised by a dietitian or pediatrician.

▶ ROADBLOCK: Is the Switch Worth It?

Is the switch from whole to low-fat milk that much of a difference? Let's take a look at 1 cup of each and find out:

- Whole milk   150 calories   8 g fat   290 mg calcium   8 g protein
- 2% milk   120 Calories   4.5 g fat   298 mg calcium   8 g protein
- 1% milk   100 Calories   2.5 g fat   300 mg calcium   8 g protein
- Skim milk   80 Calories   0.0 g fat   300 mg calcium   8 g protein

So if your five-year-old starts drinking 1% milk instead of whole milk and typically drinks 3 cups of milk a day, he would save 150 calories a day. That may not sound like much, but if you consume 150 extra calories a day, in 23 days you have gained one extra pound. You gain a pound for every 3,500 extra calories that you consume.

150 calories × 23 days = 3,450 calories = approximately 1 pound

or

150 calories × 365 days = 54,750 calories per year

54,750 calories ÷ 3,500 calories = 15.7 pounds per year

Toddlers do not need more than 24 ounces of milk a day. Children who drink too much milk instead of other nutritious food may be at an increased risk of not getting enough iron and other nutrients.

Meat and Other Protein Foods

Protein is important for your child's growth and development. By twelve months of age, children should be eating two servings daily of foods rich in protein.

By two years of age, your child is eating more table foods. Help your child choose lean protein foods, such as chicken, fish, eggs, and legumes (beans, peas). Limit high-fat protein foods, such as meats with visible fats, high-fat lunch meats, or fried meats. Many of the foods rich in protein also tend to be rich in iron. Iron will be discussed in more detail a little later.

As Michael went through the "terrible twos," he started to throw fits about certain foods. In order to get him to eat and to make mealtime manageable, his parents cooked things until they found something he would eat. Unfortunately, this was becoming a control Michael had over his parents as he continued to demand only certain foods. To eliminate the daily struggles, Michael's parents established mealtime boundaries to include set mealtimes and a set menu with no more making of unplanned items. They also encouraged Michael to sample all of the foods. Consistency with the message and approach between his parents was what finally changed Michael's behavior.

Breads, Cereal, and Starches

This food group provides the energy your child needs to grow adequately. Between 12 and 23 months, children need six servings of this food group. By the age of two, children need only three to four servings of these foods. Note the differences in serving sizes between each of the age groups (see table).

This is a good time to introduce whole-grain breads and cereals. They are higher in fiber, which reduces the risk for heart disease later in life.

Fruits and Vegetables

This food group contains a wide variety of healthy nutrients, including important vitamins and minerals. Include four to five servings of fruits and vegeta-

COLOR	FRUITS/VEGETABLES
Red	Tomatoes, pink grapefruit, watermelon
Red/purple	Red and blue grapes, blueberries, strawberries, prunes, cranberries, plums, cherries, raisins, red apples, beets, eggplant, red cabbage, red peppers
Orange	Mangoes, cantaloupe, apricots, pumpkin, winter squash, acorn squash, sweet potatoes, carrots
Orange/yellow	Oranges, tangerines, yellow grapefruit, lemon, lime, peaches, papaya, nectarines, pineapple
Yellow/green	Honeydew, kiwi, spinach, collards, mustard or turnip greens, corn, green peas, avocado, green beans, green peppers, yellow peppers, cucumber, romaine lettuce, zucchini
Green	Broccoli, brussels sprouts, cabbage, kale, bok choy
White/green	Pears, green grapes, garlic, chives, mushrooms, onions, leeks, celery, asparagus, artichoke, endive, cauliflower

Source: Adapted from the UCLA Center for Human Nutrition's Color Code System for Fruits and Vegetables.

bles each day. Try to include fruits and vegetables of different colors to ensure that your child gets the full array of vitamins and nutrients needed for growth and development.

Challenge your family to eat a rainbow of colors each week.

Important Nutrients for the Pre-K Set

Healthy children can get the nutrients they need by eating a variety of foods from all the food groups. Some key nutrients to consider during the toddler and pre-K ages:

- **Calcium** helps build strong bones. Children can meet their daily needs for calcium from milk, cheese, and yogurt.
- **Iron** helps blood carry oxygen to all parts of the body. Children who do not get enough iron in their diet may develop anemia, which means the blood has too little iron. If left untreated, iron-deficiency anemia may lead to behavioral or learning problems. These may not be reversible, even with later iron supplementation. Foods rich in iron include meats, beans, some vegetables, and iron-fortified breakfast cereals.
- **Vitamin A** helps preserve and improve eyesight. Foods rich in vitamin A include carrots, sweet potatoes, spinach, squash, and liver.
- **Vitamin C** helps build strong bones, cartilage, and connective tissue. It also helps absorb iron in the body. Many fruits and vegetables contain vitamin C, including oranges, strawberries, cantaloupe, and broccoli.
- **Vitamin D,** with the help of calcium, helps form strong bones and teeth. Vitamin D is found in milk fortified with vitamin D. Also, the body makes vitamin D when exposed to sunlight.

For a description of other vitamins and nutrients beneficial for your child's health, see Chapter 4.

You may feel that it might be easier to give your child a daily multivitamin, especially if you are strapped for time or have a picky eater. It is much healthier for your child to get all of the necessary vitamins and minerals from a well-balanced diet of foods. Vitamins and minerals found in foods, especially in fruits and vegetables, are better absorbed by the body than vitamins and minerals in a multivitamin tablet. Also, there are other nutrients found in foods that you will not find in a multivitamin tablet. For example, fruits and vegetables are rich in fiber.

► HELPFUL HINT: **Pleasing the Picky Eater**

If your child is a picky eater, especially in the fruit and vegetable department, try to present foods in different and fun ways. For example, try some of these tasty treats:

- Use low-fat dips or yogurt to dunk fresh fruit.
- Add vegetables to pizza, soups, stir-fry, or casseroles.
- Make a fruit smoothie, add fruit to cereal.
- Create a fruit or vegetable kebab.
- Make a fun arrangement on your child's plate.
- Serve foods on entertaining paper plates that your child picks out.

You also must act as a positive role model by practicing healthy eating habits in front of your child.

Juice

Although 100 percent fruit juice may sometimes be considered a fruit choice, juice should be limited to no more than 4–6 ounces a day. Most juice has less nutritional value than the fruit it comes from and has high amounts of sugar that may contribute to obesity as well as cause tooth decay. In addition, by offering juice, you may be suppressing your child's appetite for more nutritious foods. If the juice does not contain 100 percent real fruit juice, it probably has sugar added. If the beverage contains only 5 percent or 10 percent real fruit juice, consider choosing another drink. These drinks with low fruit juice content have sugar added for flavoring and minimal vitamins or minerals. While it is okay to give your child 100 percent fruit juice sometimes, he will receive more vitamins and minerals if he eats the actual fruit. Fresh fruits contain fiber, which aids in the feeling of fullness and helps to regulate bowel movements.

Fats and Oils

Fats and oils, such as butter, margarine, shortening, and lard, also should be limited for this age group. Instead, most of your child's fat sources should come from nuts (assuming no allergies) and vegetable oils, like olive oil or peanut oil. Fast foods tend to be high in fat, especially saturated fat. Keep in mind that all the fats have the same amount of calories and should be used sparingly.

► ROADBLOCK: **Eating Out with Toddlers**

Let's take a look at some healthier options you can make at fast-food restaurants:

INSTEAD OF	TRY
Fried chicken sandwich	Grilled chicken or fish sandwich
Sausage biscuit	Pancakes
Loaded baked potato	Baked potato with vegetables (instead of cheese, butter, or sour cream)
French fries or Tater Tots	Salad with fat-free dressing
Onion rings	Fresh fruit
Fried chicken tenders	Low-fat deli sandwich on wheat bread or pita
Macaroni and cheese	Pasta with spaghetti sauce
Whole milk or soda	Low-fat milk or water

Beware of Food Allergies

When introducing new foods, do so one at a time and watch for signs of food allergies, like rash, upset stomach, or difficulty breathing. Food allergens are likely to be found in:

- eggs
- wheat
- peanuts (including peanut butter)
- tree nuts: walnuts, pecans
- fish
- shellfish
- milk
- soy

Susan, a working mother with two children under the age of five, knows how important it is to give her children a healthy balanced meal in the evening. She organizes her meals in advance of her grocery shopping so that she is able to purchase some convenience food items with some fresh items to help expedite dinner preparations. Tonight she is having hamburger patties that she portioned and seasoned last night, with a frozen vegetable medley and boiled potatoes that she cut up the night before. This enables her family to get the benefit of fresh products and does not require too much preparation time to get her meal complete in a timely manner. Susan is on the ROAD to success.

Communicating About and Encouraging Healthy Weight

Social and Emotional Development Related to Nutrition

If you have a toddler, you have probably noticed that she has become a picky eater, even refusing to eat foods that she used to love . . . or so you thought. Don't get discouraged.

Continue offering these foods, as well as new ones. If you stop offering new foods, your child may not get the variety and diversity of foods she needs. Also, your child will never have the opportunity to start liking the new food if you never give her another chance to try.

According to the American Academy of Pediatrics, toddlers may need to be exposed to a food as many as fifteen times before they accept it. Do not assume that your child will never like foods she initially disliked.

Allow your child to touch, smell, feel, and taste the food as often as she likes (or doesn't like!). This is the age of exploration, so allow your child to experiment with the five senses. This may help your child feel more familiar with the food and eventually more comfortable about eating it. Don't worry about proper table manners at this stage. You have plenty of time to teach them later.

Toddlers are unpredictable. They may eat one food one day and refuse it the next. They may eat everything offered on one day and very little the next. Do not be too concerned that your toddler is not eating enough. Just make sure that you offer healthy foods and have them available, and help them understand the reasons behind choosing certain foods over others.

Parents' Responsibility

Children are unpredictable in the amounts and types of foods they eat, but they generally eat enough food to meet their nutritional needs.

It is critical to remember that it is your responsibility to keep on the ROAD to help your toddler get a good start to healthy eating. Toddlers are very aware of the environment around them and what you are doing and eating. So be sure that you are modeling healthy eating habits at this young age. To make sure your child's nutritional needs are met, you must be the one who chooses the foods and their method of preparation. Make sure that you organize and plan healthy meals and snacks. Remember, being firm about food choices is an important aspect of parenting. Parents also must have available developmentally appropriate and healthy food at scheduled meal- and snacktimes. Also make sure that the foods you serve facilitate the development of appropriate eating skills and the use of appropriate tools for feeding.

Many studies have shown that children learn to regulate their own cues for hunger and for feeling full. This is called *self-regulation* and is important for developing a natural sense of when to stop eating. However, according to Leann Birch and Jennifer Fisher, parents' feeding practices can influence their children's response to meal size.

When parents control their children's meal size or force their children to eat, rather than allowing them to focus on their internal hunger cues, children's ability to regulate their meal size decreases. This is considered one reason that some children are not able to judge appropriate portion sizes or to stop eating until they are overly full.

Best Behaviors

Schedule Mealtimes and Snacktimes

It is important for children to understand that there is a schedule when it comes to meals and snacks. A schedule enables them to have specific expectations about when food is served, where it will be served, and at what time.

Toddlers and preschoolers respond well to structure. They usually need three meals and two or three snacks between meals. Meals and snacks should be spaced apart so that your child is not too full or too hungry before or after eating. Also, you should set a specific time limit for eating so that your child knows to complete the meal within this time frame; usually 20–30 minutes is recommended. Organizing meals can create opportunities for maximizing healthy eating.

Do not allow grazing of food or sugary liquids throughout the day. If your child grazes for food during the day, he or she may give you a hard time eating the nutritious foods you offer for meals and snacks. He or she also will feel in control of the feeding schedule, which eventually becomes troublesome.

▶ ROADBLOCK: Is My Child a "Grazer"?
Here are some strategies to try if your child tends to graze all day long. Remember, this includes drinking juice or milk, even in a sippy cup.

- Divert the urge to eat or nibble with an activity. Turn on music and sing a song together. Keep your child active with games and toys. Do an activity together, whether it's chores or fun.
- Make sure your child eats well at mealtime so he or she isn't hungry between times and has an appetite when a meal is served. It is okay for your child to get hungry.
- Offer water if your child is thirsty.

Why should you avoid letting your child graze all day? A child will not feel hunger cues and learn to manage them. Bad habits will set in too early, and it is surprising how fast the calories add up, too.

Favorite Snacks for the Pre-K Set
Here are some quick and easy snack ideas for you to try with your toddler or preschooler. You'll like them, too!

- English muffin pizza with pineapple or tomato slice, mushrooms, or other veggies.
- Baked potato with chili beans or broccoli and cheese.
- Waffle topped with fresh fruit (choose fruits that are in season).
- Tortilla folded in half with melted cheese, beans, vegetables, or chicken. Use a mild salsa to dip in.
- Spread cream cheese or hummus on a tortilla, add grated vegetables plus lettuce, roll it up, and slice it into 1-inch pieces.
- Pita bread or hot dog bun with tuna salad.
- Yogurt topped with fruit and cereal.
- Raw vegetables cut into slices or sticks with a yogurt dip. (Mix your favorite dry salad dressing mix into plain yogurt to make a great-tasting low-fat dip!)
- Sliced apples (or carrots sticks and celery) dipped in peanut butter.
- Spread fruit-flavored yogurt on a graham cracker square, top it with a second square, and wrap them in plastic wrap and freeze.
- Fruit smoothie made with yogurt.
- Peanut butter, jelly, and sliced banana sandwich.
- Home-made trail mix: cereals, dried fruit, yogurt-covered raisins, nuts, and coconut.
- Frozen fruit on a stick.
- Fruit kebab.
- String popped popcorn with minimarshmallow and dried fruit (raisins, cranberries, apricots, or cherries).

Tools for Toddlers

Sitting in a chair at the table encourages positive family meals. A child has an easier time eating when sitting in a high chair or booster seat that places him or her at the correct height for eating.

Provide child-size utensils with short handles and forks with dull tines. Dishes and plates need to have a curved edge so food is easier to scoop up. Child-size utensils, cups, and plates not only help encourage eating but also help to develop your child's fine-motor skills.

Keys to Healthy Eating Habits

- Offer nonfood rewards: smiles, hugs, kisses, stickers, reading time, playtime, or a walk to the park.
- Avoid using food as a tool to bribe your child to eat other food, especially dessert.
- Offer nutrient-rich meals and snacks.
- Stay away from empty calories that are low in nutrients, like chips, cookies, juices, and sugary drinks.
- Sit down for meals as a family, without any distractions from the TV or phone.

Overcoming Picky Eating

"Yuck, I hate that!" may bring on the panicked feeling that your child won't consume adequate vitamins and minerals to keep him healthy and growing appropriately for his age. If you are not careful, this could be the beginning of a power struggle. You now start the begging, "Please, just for me, one bite," or the bribing, "If you take two small bites you can have dessert." Mealtime becomes a battle of wills rather than a time to enjoy and look forward to. None of these approaches works and ultimately your child wins control. You may even find yourself becoming a short-order cook just to get him to eat something.

What *does* work is remembering to stay on the right ROAD as a parent: **R**ole-modeling, **O**rganizing and planning while making healthy foods **A**ccessible and available and your child's responsibility, **D**eciding whether and how much to eat. If you don't establish the rules and parameters during mealtime, how will your child learn?

It is normal for children to have "food jags." They are part of being a toddler or preschooler and emerge when they want to show their independence and be assertive. Don't give up simply because your tiny tot is acting finicky. Here are some additional ideas to help with picky eaters:

- Make sure your child has his or her own dish, cup, and utensils.
- Involve your child in meal preparation and setting the table.
- Let your child choose and use a lunch box even if he or she is not in school.
- Introduce a new food by serving it along with your child's favorite food.
- Make food into fun shapes like animals. Use cookie cutters for creative shapes.
- Make mini–meat loaf in a cupcake pan when you are making a larger meat loaf for the family (or minipizzas!)

- Have your child make a place mat by decorating both sides of a piece of paper (18"×13"), then have it laminated. Your child may buy in better if he or she feels some ownership in the eating process.

These suggestions will help your child feel more involved in the eating process and excited about some of the special meals and treats.

▶ ROADBLOCK: Keep on Trying
If your child rejects a new food, try again and again:

- Try a new food along with a familiar food.
- Don't force-feed. Eating should be a positive experience, so let your child decide whether to eat and how much.
- Set a good example. If you make a face at a food or refuse to eat it yourself, then your child is likely to do the same.

Baby Bottle Tooth Decay / Sippy Syndrome

"Baby bottle tooth decay" is another name for early childhood caries, or cavities, a very common chronic disease among children in the United States. Caries usually occur in children who are frequently exposed to liquids containing sugar, soda, Kool-Aid, fruit juice, and even milk and formula. The sugar in these drinks allows bacteria in the mouth to produce acids that cause cavities and can destroy the tooth. The Academy of General Dentistry points out that "the long-term and regular use of sippy cups or bottles, past the age of one, with sugary drinks puts children's growing teeth at increased risk for decay."

Don't put your child to bed with the bottle or sippy cup, and prevent your child from constantly sipping on sugary liquids throughout the day.

Another potential problem with sippy cups may be that they disrupt speech development. Some speech pathologists believe that sippy cups prolong sucking and slurping, when a toddler should be swilling and gulping from a cup. These simple actions do more than simply make your child look grown up at the table. They are related to how the mouth and its muscles naturally develop. Drinking from a sippy cup for too long, instead of using a regular cup, can produce a lazy tongue, which can affect the way a toddler pronounces certain sounds, at least temporarily. Drinking from a cup is a developmental milestone.

Grocery Shopping with Your Child

Grocery shopping is a great opportunity for teaching your child and making learning fun because everything you buy can be a teaching tool. Here are some examples of how you can get your child involved in grocery shopping, based on his or her age and ability:

- Compare colors of produce: brown potato versus orange sweet potato, red apples versus green apples.
- Look at sizes of items: large cabbage versus small Brussels sprouts or tomatoes and cherry tomatoes.
- Look at shapes: carrot versus cantaloupe.
- Feel the texture of cucumbers versus kiwi.
- Older children might be interested in looking at the numbers on the scales and how much things weigh.
- Give your child the opportunity to choose, such as between two healthy cereals.

Childcare and Preschool Considerations

Center-based childcare has steadily increased. Approximately twelve million American children five years old or younger are in some form of childcare. This makes it important to consider what your child is consuming while being cared for by others. Childcare programs can help prevent and treat obesity in young children in several ways.

The number of obese children has increased dramatically over the last thirty years. Approximately 10 percent of children two to five years of age and 15 percent of children six to eleven years of age are overweight.

Over the years, child nutrition programs have shifted their focus from prevention of dietary deficiencies (such as iron) to promoting healthier food choices that prevent disease and promote proper growth and good health.

Based on these trends, the American Dietetic Association recommends that childcare programs provide well-balanced meals and snacks that meet the Dietary Guidelines for Americans developed by the USDA. These meals and snacks should provide child-size portions, be appetizing, and offer adequate servings from each of the food groups. Children need daily fruits, vegetables, whole grains, lean meat or meat alternates, and, after age two, low-fat dairy products. Children two years and older should be offered food every two to three hours during the active part of their day. A child's stomach is small, plus his or her energy needs can fluctuate. By offering snacks along with regular meals, your child will be more likely to meet his or her energy needs through the day.

Childcare and preschool menus should meet children's specific nutrient needs, according to the Dietary Reference Intakes (National Center for Health

Statistics). This means that children in daycare programs for four to seven hours should receive a minimum of one-third of their daily nutrients, whereas children in programs for more than seven hours should receive one-half to two-thirds of their daily nutrient needs. Calories are not the issue. Many snacks and meals contain plenty of fat and sugar. The main goal is to make certain that children have the right foods that provide important minerals and other nutrients such as iron, zinc, and magnesium. Deficiencies in these nutrients have been linked to developmental delays in children in this age group.

Childcare programs should balance nutrient and energy needs with each child's age and physical activity level. For every hour of inactivity (watching TV, playing video or computer games, or reading), a child should have ten minutes of physical activity, and this should apply seven days a week.

You need to be involved in the food served in your child's daycare. The ADA 2006 FITS study shows that families can influence their children's dietary habits at school, which is the upside. The downside is that most parents are unaware of the nutrition program at their child's daycare and the important part it plays in eating habits. Parents and childcare staff must work together to help children learn and develop good eating habits. Children also need to eat in a positive environment to help them develop their social skills at home and away from home.

Nutrition education and training for staff and families should be ongoing. According to an ADA position paper on childcare, about half of caregivers at childcare centers have no knowledge of appropriate serving sizes or of the nutrients provided by food sources. For example, juice or fruit juice mix is frequently substituted for milk, which decreases the calcium and vitamin D that are needed for bone growth and development.

Caregivers should understand the basics of planning and serving healthy meals and snacks. Through training, registered dietitians would be able to assist with menu planning and nutritional information. They could train food service workers as well as caregivers.

Nutrition education to children while in childcare programs also provides a link to the families who may need help implementing healthful food habits. A dietitian can help with age-appropriate nutrition education for parents through daycare programs or via a pediatrician. Many organizations provide free nutrition education material for parents and caregivers.

▶ HELPFUL HINT: Check Your Child's Menu
Ask your childcare program:

1. Do the meals meet established nutritional requirements and are they approved by a dietitian?
2. Are menus posted?

3. Are desserts served?
4. How many and what type of snacks do you serve?
5. What beverages do you serve?
   a. 100% juice? If so, how much?
   b. Whole or reduced-fat milk?

Physical Activity

Your child needs physical activity every day. Physical activity helps promote healthy weight and optimal bone health. According to the National Association for Sport and Physical Education, "Becoming physically active early in life is essential because it increases the chances that infants and young children will learn to move skillfully, ensures healthy development, and lessens the chance of developing sedentary lives."

The American Academy of Pediatrics recommends that television, video, and DVD time be limited to a maximum of two hours per day. Children do not need their own television, so be smart and keep it out of their bedrooms.

One study recommends that toddlers need at least 30 minutes and preschoolers need at least 60 minutes of structured physical activity daily. While they should be getting this at daycare, try to spend outdoor or active time with them too when they are with you at home, on the weekends, holidays, and summer. After all, you are still their most important role model, even if they're attending daycare.

Get Active on Your Preschooler's Level

Try some of these physical activites. Your youngster won't even realize it's exercise!

- Play Simon Says to combine different types of walks and runs (marching, hopping, jumping).
- Dance to music, songs, and nursery rhymes.
- Play chase.
- Do "Head, Shoulders, Knees, and Toes."
- Play horse by encouraging your toddler to gallop.
- Take family walks.

Setting Your Toddler and Pre-K Feeding Goals

Now try creating your personalized goals for your toddler or preschool youngster. Some sample goals:

- Each day after we get home from work/childcare, I will offer my child fresh fruit for a snack.
- This week I will purchase 2% milk for our family now that John is three years old.
- We will let our four-year-old drink from a cup every night at dinner and not give a sippy cup.

Fiction: I shouldn't worry about weight in my preschooler because a chubby child is a healthy child.

Fact: Overeating in the early years is at the root of obesity. Studies show that children who enter pre-K or school overweight are likely to gain significantly more weight after entering school.

To help your youngster stay fit, don't put him through a strict exercise regime. At younger ages, normal child's play *is* exercise. Parents can play actively with their child too—with a ball, a dog, or any outdoor activity.

Fiction: Of course my toddler carries juice around all day in her sippy cup—children need fluids. Experts recommend they drink as many as 6 to 8 glasses a day.

Fact: Juices contain significant amounts of sugar, so your child will take in too many "empty" calories if she drinks all that juice. Encourage your child to drink water by putting only water in her cup, then have her finish her drink, either sitting or standing in one place. Otherwise, she'll form the habit of walking around with a drink all the time, which isn't necessary and could lead to problems later in life.

7

• • •

Action Is Everything
in Grade School

As children enter their school-age years, they become more independent. They are busy learning reading and arithmetic, as well as the behaviors that will help them fit in with their friends. They also observe and imitate the behaviors of parents and family members and begin to identify more with gender roles.

Take a few minutes to read and answer the questions below to assess how far along the ROAD to success you and your family are.

Where Are You on the ROAD to Providing Healthy Intake for Your Grade-School Child?

YES **NO** *Check YES or NO to answer the following questions:*

☐ ☐ Does your child like to eat whole grains?

☐ ☐ Does your child enjoy trying new foods?

☐ ☐ Do you and your family eat a healthy breakfast every morning?

☐ ☐ Do you provide basic, balanced nutrition in proper portions at home?

☐ ☐ Are meal- and snacktimes consistent and regular?

☐ ☐ Are healthy food choices available and accessible in your home?

☐ ☐ Does everyone in the family avoid making negative comments about each other's weight?

☐ ☐ Do the children help with preparing meals, planning, and shopping for groceries?

☐ ☐ Is school lunch money limited to only the amount needed for that day?

☐ ☐ Is your weekend eating pattern the same as the weekdays?

☐ ☐ Do you play/exercise as a family several times each week?

☐ ☐ Do you avoid eating in front of the television?

_____ *How many yes answers did you have?*

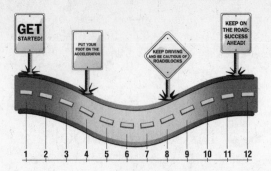

If you scored between 1 and 4, it is time to get your foot on the accelerator and focus on those small changes. If you scored between 5 and 8, you are on the ROAD to better health, but watch out for those roadblocks. If you scored between 9 and 12, use the tips in this chapter to refine and improve your goals or decisions.

Healthy Growth and Development

The number of children between six and eleven who are overweight in the United States has more than tripled since the 1970s. Because human genetic makeup could not possibly change that quickly, this rise in weight gain must be related to what children are eating and how much less they are moving. The American Dietetic Association reports that children who are overweight at this age are much more likely to become obese as adults.

What Is "Normal"?

After the rapid growth in infancy and before the growth spurts of adolescence, the school-age years represent a time of slower growth. Children at this age vary greatly in their body shapes and height. While "normal" weight can depend on many factors, generally, a normal weight range for children ages six to eleven years is 43 to 80 pounds, with no major differences between boys and girls. Children at this age should gain about ⅓ pound per month, or about 4 to 5 pounds a year, as long as they are also growing taller.

Appendix C shows growth charts for boys and girls ages two to twenty. You can use them to plot your child's weight, height, and BMI (see Appendix B) to see how he or she compares to others the same age. More important, you can follow your child's personal growth trend and visually identify any rapid gains in weight.

Important Nutrients and Portions

If the old saying "You are what you eat" applies to typical American children ages six to eleven, then they are generally composed of lots of added sugar and saturated (heart-clogging) fat. Instead of those ingredients, children at this age should be eating more fiber, calcium, iron, vitamin A, and vitamin C—in other words, whole grains, fruits, vegetables, and low-fat dairy products.

A balanced meal typically consists of a protein (meat, fish, egg, or beans), a starch/grain (bread, noodles, cereal, rice, or potato), a vegetable and/or a fruit (the brighter the color, the better), and a dairy (milk or yogurt). Make sure to include daily sources of fiber from whole fruits, vegetables, and grain products. (See Chapter 3 for more information on nutrients in specific food groups.) As children grow, it's important to adjust serving sizes for their age too. Use this table as a guide to the proper daily amount of each food group.

SCHOOL AGE CHILDREN TO ADOLESCENTS

Food Groups and Number of Daily Servings	Age 9–13 Years	Age 14–18 Years
Milk and Milk Products	**3 cups/day**	**3 cups/day**
Low-fat or fat-free milk or milk products	**1 cup =** 1 cup of milk or yogurt, 1½ ounces of a neutral cheese, 2 ounces of processed cheese, ⅓ cup of shredded cheese	
Meat and Other Protein Foods	**5 ounces/day**	**5–6 ounces/day**
Includes beef, chicken, pork, poultry, fish, eggs, peanut butter, and legumes	**1 ounce of meat =** 1 ounce of beef, poultry, or fish, ¼ cup cooked beans, 1 egg, 1 tablespoon peanut butter, ½ ounce of nuts	
Breads, Cereals, and Starches	**5–6 ounces/day**	**6–7 ounces/day**
Includes whole-grain breads, infant and cooked cereals, rice, pasta, ready-to-eat cereals. Half of all starches should be whole grains	**1 ounce =** 1 slice whole-grain bread, ½ cup cooked cereal, rice or pasta, 1 cup dry cereal	
Fruits	**1½ cup/day**	**1½–2 cups/day**
Includes one source of vitamin C daily (citrus fruits and juices, strawberries) and one source of	**1 cup =** 1 cup of fruit or 100% fruit juice, ½ cup of dried fruit (limit juice to 4–6 ounces of juice/day)	

(continued)

SCHOOL AGE CHILDREN TO ADOLESCENTS (continued)

Food Groups and Number of Daily Servings	Age 9–13 Years	Age 14–18 Years
vitamin A every other day (dark green and yellow fruits, melons)		
Vegetables *Includes one source of vitamin C daily (broccoli, tomatoes, and potatoes) and one source of vitamin A every day (spinach, sweet potatoes, corn, squash)*	**2–2½ cups/day**	**2½–3 cups/day**
	1 cup = 1 cup of raw or cooked vegetables or vegetable juice, 2 cups of raw leafy greens	
Fats and Oils *Includes margarine, butter, oils*	**5–6 servings/day**	**6–7 servings/day**
	1 serving = 1 teaspoon oil, margarine, butter, or mayonnaise 1 tablespoon salad dressing, sour cream, or light mayonnaise	
Miscellaneous *Desserts, sweets, soft drinks, candy, jam and jelly*	**Limit to small amount, use sparingly**	

Source: Created by Texas Children's Hospital, adapted by the United States Department of Agriculture.
NOTE: One serving is equivalent to the quantity listed in each age-appropriate box.

To get your child to eat new foods that he or she does not usually like, try to balance these foods with ones that your child does enjoy. Another approach is to offer a new food when your child is hungry.

> ▶ HEALTHY HINT: **Create a Nibble Tray**
> For most working parents, the first fifteen minutes at home is when the feeding frenzy begins. To avoid the pantry grazing, put together a tray of precut fruits or vegetables the night before. Place a bowl of low-fat yogurt for a dip in the center of the tray. Put this on the table when you walk in the door and watch your child fill up on nutritious foods before dinner. Likewise, don't have chips in the pantry.

If you are worried about your child's weight, don't demand that your child stop eating at a certain point in the meal. Instead, focus more on controlling portion sizes by using preportioned snack packages (make your own or buy the preportioned 100-calorie bags) and by increasing the amount of healthier foods (those lower in fat and sugar) that he or she can eat without too much concern.

Children should not skip breakfast. Research from the Third National Health and Nutrition Examination Survey gives two very compelling reasons: improved school performance and a significantly lower BMI. The best choice for kids is low-sugar breakfast cereal. The American Dietetic Association says that children who eat breakfast almost always consume a more balanced diet overall than children who do not.

School-Age Habits and Growing Appetites

Have you ever felt like your child can eat more than you can? Today's children don't have the same eating patterns that today's adults did at the same age. The American Dietetic Association found that children, especially of school age, are eating significantly larger amounts of food and drinking many more sweet beverages than children two decades ago. This is mostly the result of portions getting larger. For example, twenty years ago an average muffin was 1½ ounces and contained 210 calories. Today, that same muffin is 4 ounces and 500 calories. Here are some more examples of food portions that have changed:

FOOD	20 YEARS AGO	TODAY
Bagel	3 inches 140 calories	6 inches 350 calories
French Fries	2.4 oz 140 calories	6.9 oz 610 calories
Soda	6.5 oz 85 calories	20 oz 250 calories

Children are definitely eating more adult-size portions, especially outside the home. This puts you in the position of making sure you provide basic, balanced nutrition in proper portions at home, because it is most likely that your child will get plenty of extra calories (from sugars and fats) outside of home, and not get the best nutrition.

Communicating About Healthy Weight

As a parent, you are responsible for the access to and availability of foods presented to your child but not the amount eaten. This was easier to control during the preschool years, but now your child will be exposed to eating new and different foods at school, friends' houses, and at other places in the community. As school-age children spend more time with friends, the likelihood of eating also increases.

You must tell your child when she is eating too much junk food and encourage her to choose healthier foods. However, you also must avoid being too pushy or domineering, as you may negatively influence your child's ability to develop good judgment for herself. Forbidding your child to have candy may cause her to hoard it when it becomes available. Instead, try to provide a positive and supportive eating relationship with your child that is neither too demanding nor permissive. Teaching your child that there are foods we eat less often versus forbidden foods is more effective.

Continue to offer nutritious meals and snacks at home and stick to regular eating times. For some children, it is helpful if healthcare professionals or non-family members encourage these behaviors as well. This is the perfect age to involve your child in fun and interactive nutrition education either in books or on the Internet.

> ▶ HELPFUL HINT: Surf the Web
> These Web sites have food and nutrition activities for children. Visit them often, as they are frequently updated with new information or activities.
>
> www.eatright.org
> www.mypyramid.gov
> www.nationaldairycouncil.org
> www.nutrition.gov

Check out more Web sites found on pages 271–272.

Age of Influence

Children choose better when they receive acceptance and guidance rather than absolutes or limits. What you teach and role-model for your child about food at a young age will shape his or her relationship with food as an adolescent and adult.

Overwhelming evidence has shown that eating habits and patterns are ingrained by the time children are about eleven years of age, or in sixth grade. It is not enough to tell children, "Eat healthy foods." These food must be available and accessible in your home. You also must be seen making the same healthy choices. If you want to a have a stronger impact on what and how your child eats, make changes and intervene as early as possible, preferably before the age of twelve. Remember that media is not always on our side. Children are continuously exposed and made susceptible to unhealthy foods by advertising. A recent report by the Institutes of Medicine urges the food industry to curtail its marketing to children. Of the more than $200 billion spent by youth on food, independent of their parents, choices are typically high-calorie, low-nutrient foods. Cartoons, cartoon characters, and colorful graphics are used to entice children to want specific foods. However, in most cases the ultimate purchasing power rests with the parents. Limiting high-calorie, low-nutrient foods is your gift to your child.

Being a good role model for your child also includes what you say. Be careful how you express your concerns about your own body image or your child's as well as your beliefs about food. Children are dieting at an earlier age, whether they need to or not. Research by Michael Maloney and colleagues demonstrated that up to 37 percent of children in grades three to six had already tried to lose weight and up to 45 percent of children wanted to be thinner. What you say about yourself, your body, and your eating influences your child even if you think he or she isn't paying attention. Research by Alison Field and associates tracking the influence of parents, peers, and the media demonstrated that children who want to look like the same-sex figures portrayed in the media are more likely to become very concerned about their weight. Additionally, children who report that their thinness was important to their fathers were more likely to be dieters.

But it can go the other way too. Negative comments about weight from family members are associated with an increased risk of being overweight. So parents, siblings, or peers calling children derogatory names in an attempt to get them to lose weight only serves to lower their self-esteem and increase their risk of obesity.

Demonstrate your concern and approval by what you do, not by what you say. The key to the ROAD to success is to eat healthy foods *with* your children—don't ask them to do what you won't yourself.

Encouraging Best Behaviors

As a parent, you have a major impact on what your child eats and how he or she feels about food. Some of the most common mistakes parents make about food and children are:

- requiring them to finish all the food on their plate
- using food as an incentive or a threat
- allowing dessert routinely
- eating irregularly scheduled meals

To counter this, focus on the good eating behaviors that follow below. Remember the ROAD.

Foundation of School-Age Mealtimes

The nutritional habits your child learns at home are likely to be the habits he or she will continue with later in life. Take your responsibility as the food provider seriously and appreciate your ability to influence your child's eating. Organize your shopping list and buy and plan nutritionally balanced meals for your child.

During the school-age years, children are still learning to accept foods, so continue to offer a large variety of new foods in addition to the usual favorites. Try to keep foods that are less nutritious out of the house, but don't become the "food police." Allowing some less nutritious food once in a while increases variety and adds excitement to meals, as long as it's not too often. Don't worry, your child has plenty of opportunities to eat favorite less nutritious foods outside the home.

Stick to regular meal- and snacktimes. That way, your child knows when he or she will be eating and won't be as tempted to eat unnecessary snacks. Also, children tend to accept the foods you offer because they are routine. Children are creatures of habit and generally learn to accept foods that other members of their family prefer, so be sure to offer lots of healthy foods like vegetables regularly when they're young—as long as you eat them too!

Snack Smart!

Most schoolchildren live for snacktime because they really need a pick-me-up between meals. Encourage and allow routine healthy snacks, and plan for them as you do for meals.

According to the American Dietetic Association, after-school and evening snacks provide at least 20 percent of children's calorie needs. This means they have fewer "available" calories for food served at mealtimes. These excess calories can promote weight gain if you and your child don't monitor snacking.

The trick to healthy snacking is not letting it ruin your appetite at mealtime and not allowing it to provide too many calories. Let your school-age child pick his or her own snacks, within reason, of course, from the list of healthy, low-calorie snacks on page 63.

Cook and Shop Together

School-age children enjoy participating in daily activities and take pride in accomplishing tasks. Have your children help you with preparing meals, planning lists, and shopping for groceries that are balanced and healthy. This encourages interest in choosing healthy foods. It also may encourage your child to be more willing to eat these healthier foods later.

Shopping and cooking together provides opportunities for you to talk about wise choices and even teach your youngster to read nutrition labels. Try to make it fun by asking challenging questions that your child may enjoy knowing the answer to.

School Lunch

Most children eat lunch at schools that have snack bars and vending machines. They also are drinking more beverages that are filled with sugar. Soft drinks are currently the leading source of added sugar in the diets of young children. According to a study by David Ludwig and colleagues, between 1989 and 1995, the amount of sugar-sweetened beverages consumed by adolescent boys increased by 8 ounces per day, resulting in increasing body weight. Although snack bars or vending machine items become a big concern in high school, most elementary schools generally do not have them, so your child may not yet have this unhealthy option at school.

In a perfect world, your child's school lunch program would have nutritionally balanced and tasty meals. Unfortunately, this is not always true and children often are tempted by unhealthy foods at school. Even if junk food isn't available, fried food often is. However, federal regulations require all school lunches served on a tray to meet minimum nutrient requirements. Many schools are becoming more and more health conscious. In Texas, for example, laws are in place to eliminate fried foods from cafeterias in public schools by 2009.

Take time to learn what foods are available to your child at school and how they are cooked. If possible, look at the school lunch menu with your child and try to guide him to healthier choices. Check out the prices too. Although you cannot control what your child chooses to eat at school, you can control how much he can buy. Don't give your child more school lunch money than he needs, as extra desserts are a temptation.

Of course, packing a healthy lunch is always a good option. Whether your child is packing a lunch or eating at school, check in with him to learn what he had to eat that day.

Eating Out and Weekends

Eating out can be a real challenge. It is almost a sure bet that when you eat out, you and your child consume more calories than you need—usually in unbalanced nutrients.

Limit your fast-food or restaurant visits, aiming for no more than once a week. When you do eat out, make sure to drink calorie-free beverages or low-fat milk and stick to proper portions or lower-fat options (see Chapter 3 for more details).

Fast-food restaurants are required to publish the nutrition content of their food online or make it available at the restaurant. Take a look and know what you and your child are eating! Aim for no more than 500 to 600 total calories per meal.

Your family's weekend eating pattern should not be different from that on weekdays. Watch out for the weekend eat-whatever-you-want mentality. This can throw off your child's eating routine and unintentionally promote weight gain. Children increase their food consumption while watching TV on the weekends. Up to one-quarter of the calories consumed by children are in front of the TV, resulting in less fruit and vegetable consumption.

Physical Activity

Exercise alone, like diet alone, is not the solution to maintaining a healthy weight, but both together can make a positive difference. Physical activity burns calories and promotes muscle tone, which in turn burns even more calories. Physical activity also provides time away from food and other cues to eat.

Two Is Better than One: Be Active Together!

Now that your child is school-age, she will not only participate in recess and physical education classes at school but also is old enough to take part in unsupervised exercise at home and around the neighborhood. Examples include cleaning the house, yard work, walking the dog, riding a bike, playing with friends, partaking in community sports teams (baseball, soccer, or swimming), or enjoying local trails and parks. Encourage your child to try different activities and choose ones that she likes.

Better yet, try these activities *with* your child as often as you can. You'll find that child is much more eager to participate if you're "playing" with her. In addition, you can arrange (or encourage) outdoor activities with your child's friends.

Don't force your child to perform activities that she doesn't like. Continue trying to find ones that interest her. Most children like at least one form of physical activity. The goal is to engage in that activity for at least 60 minutes every day. Take advantage of the daylight hours after school, on weekends, and during the summer. For tips on being active and having fun, see Chapter 4.

Limit Screen Time

Limit TV, computer, and video game time. Although your child must use the computer for homework, large amounts of screen or media time lead to an inactive body, which promotes weight gain.

The American Academy of Pediatrics recommends that children over the age of two limit television watching to no more than two hours a day. Yet a 2004 study by Dimitri Christakis and colleagues estimates that 40–48 percent of children go over this suggested amount daily.

Consider making a rule that your child must get up and move around (walk, play a sport, or clean) at least 30 minutes for every hour of screen time. This extra effort burns some calories and keeps your child active, and also gives him or her time to "come up for air" and realize there's another world beyond the screen. Additionally, it is not a good habit to let your child eat in front of the TV or computer, or even when reading a book. Make sure that these rules are imposed on everyone in the family, not just those who are overweight.

Setting Goals for Your Grade-School Child

Now try creating your personalized goals for your grade-school child. Here are some examples:

- Each time Susan watches television, I will remind her to move around or be active (walk, play a sport, or clean up) at least 30 minutes for every hour of screen time.
- We will only eat fast foods one time per week and will plan with Steven what foods are the most appropriate.
- I will send a packed lunch to school two times this week and plan the menus ahead of time.

Fiction: If I really had a weight problem, my doctor would tell me so.

Fact: Many doctors don't say much about a child being overweight. This is partly because it can be a difficult topic (some parents even get defensive and deny it's true). Also, many doctors haven't felt they had much to offer in the way of help.

Recently, doctors are being given tools to help them approach and treat patients when they see obesity. One important tactic is to teach parents to teach their children good eating habits, because the root causes of obesity may begin early in life. Healthcare providers and parents who can get control with these youngsters can help decrease the risk of obesity in later years.

8

. . .

Staying Tuned to Tweens

As your child grows and develops, the middle-school years create a unique set of concerns. Early teens are often referred to as tweens, meaning between a child and a teen. Puberty is looming in the not so distant future. As you navigate down the ROAD, see how tuned you are to your tween. Answer the following the questions to assess how far along the ROAD to success you are.

Where Are You and Your Tween on the ROAD?

YES   NO   *Check YES or NO to answer the following questions:*

☐   ☐   Have you set limits on the amount of screen time for your family?

☐   ☐   Have you allowed more decision making from your tween regarding food and fitness choices?

☐   ☐   Does your tween talk to you about weight concerns?

☐   ☐   Is your tween confident about self-appearance?

☐   ☐   Do you avoid using food as a punishment or reward for your tween?

☐   ☐   Have you set boundaries on what foods you will not provide for your tween?

☐   ☐   Are you aware of what foods are available for your tween at school?

☐   ☐   Have you talked with your tween about healthy lunch options to bring from home?

☐   ☐   Do you include your tween in food decisions?

☐   ☐   Do you encourage your tween to stay active?

☐   ☐   Do you engage in family exercise or family activity on most days of the week?

☐   ☐   Can you picture yourself as both a coach and a fan of your tween?

_____   *How many yes answers did you have?*

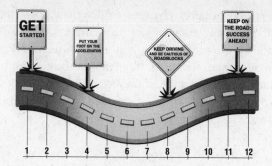

If you scored between 1 and 4, it is time to get your foot on the accelerator and focus on those small changes. If you scored between 5 and 8, you are on the ROAD to better health, but watch out for those roadblocks. If you scored between 9 and 12, use the tips in this chapter to refine and improve your goals or decisions.

Puberty: Friend or Foe?

There's no calendar or time line that predicts exactly when everyone will experience the same part of puberty, but certain changes in body composition do affect everyone at some point.

Boys' bodies grow up (height) and out (weight) at about the same time. Between the ages of ten and seventeen, muscle mass can double for teenage boys. Their most rapid gains in height and weight occur between the ages of fifteen and seventeen.

For girls, peak growth typically occurs between the ages of eleven and fourteen. Their peak height growth occurs about six months before peak weight growth. In the course of normal puberty, girls get taller first, followed by an accelerated weight gain—girls grow "up" and then "out."

The time between growing "up" and "out"—about six months—can be a time of anxiety, with comments like, "I'm getting so fat." When it comes to body image, the average girl likes getting taller but does not like the normal weight gain that follows. But it's the increasing levels of hormones that cause girls to add on this "good fat," which is part of what makes a girl a girl.

Physical Change

Growth is different for boys and girls during this early adolescent stage. Although the most rapid growth for girls happens between ages eleven and fourteen years, some may experience these physical changes as early as nine. Girls start having periods at an average age of twelve and a half years. Because girls may start growth and puberty changes earlier than boys, their most rapid period of growth is usually complete by sixteen years of age. Boys have their most rapid period of growth beginning at about fifteen and go through this exciting phase later than the girls. Remember those eighth-grade dances where the girls towered over most of the boys? During this period of life, the difference in growth and development can make tweens feel different, while so many of them are just trying to fit in.

> *Maria is a fourteen-year-old girl who first started her period at age eleven, which is earlier than most girls. At twelve she was the tallest girl in her class and was self-conscious about her height. As her friends started to grow, Maria started the second stage of the physical changes of tweens. She began to fill out. She was concerned that she was different from her friends and that she was fat. Maria's mother reassured her that her growth patterns were very normal and that not everyone grows at the same time.*

Calorie balance is important in these critical years. Although growth may be rapid, most children in this age group usually have no difficulty getting adequate calories. This is also the time when many tweens begin to decrease their physical activity. Computers, television, text messaging, and telephones have replaced roller skates.

Normal weight gain for your child depends on height changes. An adolescent who is tall for his or her age would be expected to have a higher rate of weight gain, and a shorter adolescent for his or her age should not be gaining as much weight. You can ask your child's doctor or dietitian to help determine a normal amount of weight gain for your child during early adolescence.

Psychological Development

As your child adjusts to physical changes, her thinking about the world around her changes as well. The hormonal changes that come along with puberty may greatly impact the moods of your child between the ages of eleven and fourteen. One day she is happy, the next day moody. The age at which your child goes through this stage of development can also affect mood as well as self-esteem. Some researchers say that early-maturing girls are more likely to have low self-esteem and poorer self-image than late-maturing girls. This may be due to hormonal changes that occur with the start of puberty. When a young adolescent notices that her body is growing, she may become dissatisfied with what she sees. It is important to remember that your child will likely be more emotional about the body changes if she starts the puberty process earlier than her friends.

Younger children think in black-or-white or all-or-none terms. Your tween is beginning to think in a more complex manner, consider consequences, create alternatives, and understand the views of others. Thinking in this manner may start around age eleven, but it takes years to develop fully. Between the ages of eleven and fourteen, your child will be able to process more complex ideas, but most adolescents show the majority of complex reasoning when they are around seventeen.

Another psychological change that begins during early adolescence is your child's view of himself or herself. Your early adolescent child may base his or her identity on the views of family or friends that will affect how you should address any weight-related concerns.

Communicating About Healthy Weight

Adolescents are typically (over)concerned with their looks. Most experience a heightened sensitivity to the opinions of their peers and family members, so knowing when to intercede is critical. You must learn how to be sensitive to your child's emotional needs while still being able to communicate about health and health-related issues.

Teasing Tweens

Studies suggest that teens who are teased about their weight by their parents are more likely to experience dissatisfaction with their bodies if the teasing comes from the father and more likely to be depressed if the teasing comes from the mother.

Remember the Sensitivity of the Younger Adolescent

Carolyn is an eleven-year-old who has consistently remained in the 95th percentile on her growth charts. She received a recent diagnosis of hyperinsulinemia and obesity. Her mother is thin and works hard to stay in shape. She explains her daily workout routine and healthy eating regimen, and is quick to pass judgment on Carolyn's "lack of willpower" when it comes to "dieting" and her constant "lazy" behaviors. Carolyn shrinks in her chair with a look of disappointment, knowing she will never live up to her mother's expectations.

As a parent, knowing when to let go and when to assert your authority can be difficult. As your child reaches the early adolescent or tween years, these boundaries go from black and white to a fuzzy gray somewhere in between.

Early adolescence is the time when your child is starting to gain his independence and to discover who he is as an individual. As the saying goes, "The apple doesn't fall far from the tree," but trying to mold your child into a smaller version of yourself may not offer the appropriate support he needs. Allow your tween to find what is unique about him. Take pride in knowing that these distinctive qualities are stepping-stones to becoming the amazing individual you are in the process of raising. Supporting your child also means continuing your role as a parent, so you must still set appropriate boundaries without monitoring your child's every move.

Encouraging, Not Monitoring

While trying to discuss Carolyn's eating habits and average food intake, her mother insists on reporting all of the "wrong foods" Carolyn eats on a daily basis. As her mother lists every chip and cookie Carolyn has consumed, one begins to envision a shiny badge hanging on the right pocket of Carolyn's mother's blouse emblazoned with the words FOOD POLICE.

A study by Leann Birch and Jennifer Fisher noted that restrictive parental behavior may actually backfire and encourage the preference for high-fat, calorie-rich foods by disrupting the normal hunger and fullness clues that we are born with. You can control what you bring into the home, but policing food is not the best strategy for long-term weight control.

Tweens cannot drive themselves to the grocery store, which makes you responsible for the food choices in the home. Yes, your adolescent is old enough to open a bag or box of food, or put something in the oven or microwave, but you are the provider of the kinds of foods allowed in the house.

> ▶ ROADBLOCK: Mentoring Versus Monitoring
>
> Rather than taking on the impossible role of being the constant food monitor, educate your child on how to make healthier choices. Tweens still seek approval from their parents, and visiting a nutrition Web site together might be a fun and new way of communicating the eat healthy message. MyPyamid.gov is a great site for you and your tween. Stock the cupboards with foods you know will allow your child to grow into a healthy adult, rather than chips, cookies, candy, and soda that don't provide the nutrients needed for growth and development.

This does not mean that junk foods are absolutely forbidden. You do not need to constantly drill the good-food, bad-food rules into your child's head. As you supply the healthier options more often, and still allow small amounts of the foods most kids love that aren't the healthiest choices, you can show your tween how to balance all types of foods to achieve a healthy, well-rounded diet.

Set an example by making healthy choices yourself at both meal- and snacktimes. Know that although your child is becoming more independent, she always will look to you as a role model to guide her along the way. Children are like sponges—they soak up every habit you pass along, including how you eat. Do you find yourself constantly answering, "Why can't we have chips and sodas in the house?" As your child matures, she will eventually understand that you made these choices in order to encourage a healthy lifestyle and teach healthy habits. Your tween can begin to understand that although chips and soda taste good, it does not mean they are good for you.

Taste buds don't know what they are missing. If you never drank sodas growing up, you probably don't crave them now. If fruits and vegetables were a staple as a child, you most likely find them important to include in your diet as an adult. As a parent, stand your ground with the healthier choices you are making. Taking care of the health of your family is your job.

Knowing When to Intercede

John is twelve years old and extremely overweight. There is a family history of diabetes, and both parents are overweight as well. John's typical daily diet includes the following:

- *high-sugar cereal with whole milk, 16 ounces of orange juice, cinnamon roll, and fruit punch (breakfast at school)*
- *nachos, ice cream sandwich, and a 20-ounce sports drink (lunch at school)*
- *chips and cookies and whatever else he can find in the "snack drawer"*
- *fast food on most nights*

John's parents are very worried about the possibility of him becoming a diabetic, but they say that trying to make him change his eating habits would only cause a "constant battle." John's mother has tried to get rid of the snack drawer many times, but John throws a fit when the chips and cookies he loves are not readily accessible. John sits through the doctor's appointment with his arms crossed and a smug look on his face, knowing he has his parents wrapped around his finger. As they start to discuss the changes that need to be made, John's only response is a two-letter word he knows all too well, "NO."

Parents often fall into the habit of giving in to their children's wants rather than their needs. Although tweens are gaining a lot more independence, you are still the parent and your job includes setting limits and boundaries. Because you are the provider, you have the responsibility of coming up with the appropriate restrictions, even when it comes to foods.

Giving in to a fit over food choices, knowing that your overweight child is on the verge of a life-threatening disease, is never a good idea. Do not feel guilty for taking care of your child's health needs. You can support a conversation with your child by remaining the parent, being authoritative but not authoritarian, and having dialogue about health needs. You can start by asking him for his thoughts and show your support with a listening ear and your ability to assist in brainstorming solutions. You can also take the first step by involving your child in the process. Ask which foods are his favorites and which he eats just because they are there. Instead of eliminating his favorite snacks, purchase them in single-serving bags to control portions, look for reduced-fat versions, and gradually change the snacks available at home.

Snacks should be structured at specific times and serve the same purpose as a meal but in a smaller version. Snacks are needed to support the important calorie and nutrient needs of a growing adolescent. Make snacks filling enough to get your tween to the next meal, but don't have an open snack policy so that he is constantly in and out of the kitchen after school until dinnertime.

If you know your child will be at home alone in the afternoon, a discussion the night before about what is available for an afternoon snack can guide him in the right direction. Spending a few minutes after school preparing a snack will make it easier for him when he comes home. Having candy, chips, or sodas readily available but telling your child to grab an apple and peanut butter when he gets home only sets him up for failure.

▶ HELPFUL HINT: Serve Balanced Snacks
Think of a snack as a minimeal and aim for it to include at least two or three food groups. Here are some tasty snacks for tweens:

- apple slices and individual single-serve peanut butter
- string cheese and a handful of whole wheat crackers
- 2 cups light popcorn and an orange
- 1 cup raw vegetables with ¼ cup hummus or low-fat ranch dressing

Food Choices at School

You can gain control at home when it comes to your family's food choices. You know exactly what you're putting in that grocery cart, and have no doubt that your family is receiving a variety of healthy foods based on the foods you supply. But what happens when you hand your child lunch money every day and put her in charge of choosing what you hope is a well-balanced lunch?

Unfortunately, most schools continue to provide a constant supply of pizza, cheeseburgers, chicken nuggets, nachos, french fries, and fast-food restaurant options for their lunch menu. A tween with a few dollars in her pocket can suddenly become powerful. You may think she is making the healthy choices that mirror what you provide at home, but the hard truth is that their peers and their taste buds influence most adolescents. That lunch money probably is not going toward the well-balanced lunch you would prefer. Because the money for a tray lunch doesn't cover the cost of an entire fast-food meal that your child will actually purchase, your child may be arriving home quite hungry and eat everything in sight. You can counter the afternoon munchies by becoming more aware of what is provided for lunch at school. Most schools have a menu available to parents, either online or on paper. After becoming familiar with it, you can talk with your tween about what food choices are available and whether they include vending machines or a snack bar line. Discuss how to make lunch a well-balanced meal and put your money to good use.

Pack a Lunch

If you find yourself running into limited options, regain your control and discuss with your tween the idea of packing a lunch. Have your child participate in what foods you include so that he'll eat them. Make sure the packed lunch includes a variety of food groups and nutrients. A great balanced lunch could include two grains (whole wheat sandwich bread), one lean meat (2–3 ounces of turkey), one low-fat dairy (light cheese on the sandwich or a yogurt), and one fruit or vegetable serving. As long as you can keep it chilled, throw in a reduced-calorie drinkable yogurt for a sweet treat. Keep in mind, however, that if it is not "cool" to bring lunch from home, you might have to adjust what is being served at mealtimes and eat a lighter meal at night.

You can get creative. Turn a sandwich into a wrap by using a whole-grain tortilla instead of bread. Depending on how flexible your child is, you can make a side salad in a resealable bowl instead of sending the typical bag of carrots. If a microwave is available, pack a cup of soup as a side to a sandwich.

An important place to start is by asking your tween whether he prefers to use a thermal lunch box or a paper bag. Tweens tend to do what their friends are doing, and they don't want to be embarrassed by being the only one with a lunch box.

Another way to encourage a packed lunch is to know your child's circle of friends and what they are eating for lunch. In most cases, if your child's friends are bringing their own lunch, your job is going to be a lot easier.

If your tween and his friends are involved in any kind of activity or sport together, that can be a useful incentive. With sports and activities usually happening in the afternoon, appropriate consumption of foods and snacks throughout the day improves performance. Carrying foods to eat at lunch and to snack on later can encourage your child to stick with the good stuff, especially if his friends are asking to share. Many options are available for making a healthy lunch more appealing while also maintaining a better balance. Adding one or two healthy snacks along with a balanced breakfast and lunch may lead to less hunger in the afternoon. One study actually shows that obese individuals tend to consume most of their energy intake in the evening, usually skipping breakfast and lunch earlier in the day.

> ▶ **ROADBLOCK: Let's Make a Deal**
> If your tween loves the snack food line at school with the pizza and nachos and you want your child to pack a lunch, make a deal. Look at this potential roadblock as an opportunity. Organize the week by looking at the school lunch menu and allowing that favorite meal possibly two out of the five school days. Using this strategy allows your child some control while keeping the weekly plan in check.

The same study suggested that calorie consumption later in the day is more readily stored as fat, rather than utilized as energy for daily living. Therefore, eating breakfast and lunch can result in a more even distribution in calorie consumption throughout the day and may result in better portion control in the evening. However, a snack still is required after school because eating every three to four hours reduces extreme hunger and lessens the risk of overeating. The good news is that if your tween increases consumption in the middle of the day, you will find it easier to keep the afternoon snack and dinner in the proper portions.

Too Cool to Take Lunch

For adolescents, appearance is extremely important. Unfortunately, what they eat also becomes trendy, making it hard to encourage a packed lunch if no one else takes his or her lunch.

Most school cafeterias offer a hot tray lunch with a variety of food groups, a snack bar line with the usual fast-food favorites, and vending machines. Explore all of these options and use the same knowledge you would use in a restaurant. Find out what is being offered in the tray line each week and discuss likes and dislikes with your child. If he or she likes the spaghetti on the tray but not any of the sides, suggest balancing the spaghetti with low-fat milk, and throw an apple in the backpack too. This increases one food group (grain) to three groups (grain, dairy, and fruit). Remember, balance and food group variety provide an increase in satiety, or the feeling of fullness. The addition of fresh fruits and vegetables adds valuable fiber and fluid, both key components of the fullness factor.

If you're trying to help your child navigate the snack bar line, look for grilled options or lean deli sandwiches such as turkey instead of chicken strips and fries. Check whether any fruit or vegetables are served and pack them if they're not. Stay away from liquid calories, such as whole milk, fruit punch, or sports drinks. Although schools are being applauded for their recent efforts to remove sodas, most are replacing those drinks with sports drinks and fruit punches, which equally contribute to an excess consumption of empty calories. Sports drinks are of value to the competitive athlete but are not needed by others.

Physical Activity

Have you ever taken the time to analyze your day to see how much of it you spend on your feet compared to sitting down? Whether you go to school or work, are you spending a majority of the day behind a desk or in front of a computer? For most people, the answer to both of these questions is that a large portion of their day is spent being sedentary.

Technology and increased urbanization have led to fewer reasons to move significantly in the course of a normal day. This has caused a major impact on the amount of daily physical activity people perform and has contributed greatly to the obesity epidemic.

These excuses for lack of movement occur not only at home but in schools as well. As adolescents enter middle school and high school, the requirements for physical education decline. According to the Centers for Disease Control's School Health Policies and Programs Study, only 6 percent of middle and junior high schools nationwide provide daily physical education or its equivalent. Additionally, 25 percent of middle schools allow exemption from a physical education course for various reasons.

For many school-age children the result is that a major part of the day is spent sitting, followed by more sitting at home doing homework, followed by sitting in front of the TV, computer, or game screen. Until the schools kick it up a notch and require mandatory physical education for grades K through twelve, incorporating activity into the after-school routine at home becomes all the more essential.

▶ **ROADBLOCK: Does Your School Make the Grade?**
With the national trend away from mandatory physical education (PE) in schools, check on the policy in your school district. During open house and other appropriate times, inquire about the PE

curriculum. Questions to ask: How many days per week is PE? What is done? Are there any other courses such as drama that the school allows for PE credit? If PE isn't up to your standards, make these exercise opportunities available for your child.

Make Exercise a Family Choice

Emily is eleven years old and has visited the Wellness Center many times with little change in her weight. She is obese and consistently gaining weight. During her exercise portion of the visit, Emily seems to thoroughly enjoy being active and actually complains when the time comes to sit down and discuss her recent dietary and exercise habits.

Exploring what has been going on since the last visit, Emily states that she is still "not really exercising after school." When asked why, she says, "No one will exercise with me, I can't fix my bike, and I don't know how to work the treadmill"—shooting her mother a blaming look as she goes through the list of excuses. Emily's mother, who is also overweight, defensively states that she has knee pain and that "exercise is painful for her to do," but she once again "promises" to help motivate Emily to do the exercise without her. The suggestions at this visit were for Emily's mom. Fixing the bike, allowing her to bike with a friend, and purchasing a fun dance video were solutions for both Emily and her mom.

When it comes to this age group and their newfound abilities to become more independent, you may have difficulty distinguishing what should be left up to the adolescent and what you should still provide. Adolescents no longer need to hold your hand while crossing the road, but they still can't make all their choices independently or engage in all activities on their own.

When it comes to physical activity, parents serve as major role models to encourage an active lifestyle for their tweens, who usually find exercise much more enjoyable when done with a friend or family member. Exercising with your tween is a great way to hold yourself accountable, as well as enjoying some company while breaking a sweat. The more active you and your child can be throughout the day, the healthier you both will feel and become. Remember that what you are and what you role-model is what your child will become.

Performing at least 20 to 30 minutes of vigorous activity on most days is what the most recent 2005 Dietary Guidelines for Americans recommend. For weight control, this needs to increase to up to 60 minutes per day. Take 30 minutes out of the afternoon, perhaps between homework and dinner, and take a brisk walk or bike ride. Or if that's too early, go together after dinner.

Now that there are so many new ways to record your favorite TV shows, you have no excuse for an evening strapped to the couch.

Exercise isn't the only way to be active. Everyday activities can help you simply to move more throughout the day, including household chores, playing outdoors, walking the dog, riding your bike, taking stairs when you have the option, and much more.

If your tween refuses to exercise but loves screen time (including TV and computer), limit that time to less than 2 hours a day. Soon your tween will be asking you to spend some time together, and you can use that time to take a walk and talk. Decreasing screen time can be a very important first step toward a more active lifestyle.

Weekends and Activity

The biggest challenge for most people, when it comes to activity, is the weekends. Your child had a long week at school and parents have a list of chores to do. Yet you have many options for making an active weekend enjoyable. Take it upon yourself to find fun activities.

Plan your weekends to include various events that you might not normally do. Go to the park, go to the museum, hang out with friends at the pool, get some yard work or housework accomplished, or go window-shopping at the mall. In other words, fill your weekend days with movement, and save your couch time for an evening movie. You'll enjoy relaxation much more if you actually get active earlier in the day.

Weather and Activity

Rain or shine, there is no excuse for omitting activity from your life. Many activities can be done regardless of the weather. If it's too hot or rain is preventing you from your evening walk, strap on your tennis shoes and head to the mall, or stay inside and dance, dance, dance. Join the nearest gym and participate in the various indoor classes, or turn your home into your own personal gym and purchase a variety of fun exercise videos.

Another option is to find a nearby pool for hot summer days and challenge yourself to water jog or participate in a water aerobics class. If you know how to swim, lap swimming is an excellent aerobic activity. If that is not an option available, plan activities that avoid the heat of the day. A midmorning walk around the apartment complex avoids the heat in the late afternoon. There are many alternatives on bad weather days, so don't use weather as an excuse. If you have the space, try a hula-hoop contest in the garage. Switching between different activities is also a great way to avoid boredom, so take advantage of varying weather and enjoy the variety.

Your Role as a Coach and a Fan

Davis is eleven years old and has recently joined a club soccer team. He loves every minute of it and is usually the first one out on the field during each practice. The only problem is that Davis does not have the natural talents that some of his teammates have been blessed with and he is a bit overweight. His father, who is also the team's coach, grew up passionate about the sport and continues to play in a men's league. He finds his son's performance an embarrassment and is very hard on Davis with every mistake he makes.

At each game you can pick Davis's father out of the crowd, screaming until he is red in the face and threatening to take Davis off the team if he doesn't "try harder." While Davis starts the games bouncing with excitement, he usually leaves the field at the end of the game with his shoulders down and his head hanging low.

With Davis, you can see both ends of the spectrum when it comes to loving sports. Davis may not end up with an athletic scholarship in the future, but he enjoys the game. The increased physical activity is valuable to prevent further weight gain. However, his father's consistent demeaning comments eventually may lead Davis down the path of taking himself out of sports altogether. Davis may equate this experience in soccer to other exercise and never quite feel good enough to participate in any activity.

Davis's father's love of the sport and unrealistic expectations are poisoning soccer for Davis. The only way Davis can make progress at the sport is by having more constructive criticism. His father's energy would be better spent encouraging Davis to continue working toward improvement and using his obvious passion to enhance his son's abilities, perhaps spending more one-on-one time, sharing his personal talents, and molding Davis into a better player. Another alternative is to have Dad not coach his son's team.

Your role as a coach and fan for your own child is to share your support for and excitement about her different abilities. Support your tween in any sport she finds interesting and continue that support if she decides to move on to another sport. Whatever you do, be sure to get out there and practice with your child—you'll be role-modeling at the same time you're building her skill and reducing everyone's waistline.

Just because you were an all-star swimmer or loved your years on the football team does not mean your tween is going to share the same passion. Introducing her to a sport is fine, but forcing your teen to stay within that activity—just because *you* think she should love it—is not an ideal way to show you care. Putting that kind of pressure on your child can backfire, turning her against activity altogether. The goal should be to improve physical activity and lifelong health.

These are critical years for discovering passions that may become lifelong loves. By age twelve, young people are old enough to make this journey on their own, but with the appropriate guidance provided by family and friends, they find it much easier to excel in any new activity.

Setting Goals for Your Tween

Now try to create your own personalized goals with your tween. Here are some examples:

* I will review the school menu choices for the healthier options every week this month.
* I will have Jennifer pack a healthy lunch three days per week.
* This month I will create two new opportunities for after-school play.
* I will limit my time on video games to one hour a day and ride my bike for thirty minutes.

Fiction: My tween may be a little chubby, but as she grows into her teen years she'll slim down.

Fact: That was true about twenty years ago, but changes in our culture (more fatty foods, less exercise) make it difficult to slim down without doing more than just waiting. In most cases, overweight adolescents tend to remain overweight for the rest of their lives. Also, an overweight teen has an 80 percent chance of becoming obese as an adult. The name of the game is early prevention—catch it before it's too late.

9

• • •

Older Teens:
Teaching Without Telling

Becoming a young man or woman is exciting, mystifying, and—face it—downright terrifying at times. What often makes it scary is not knowing what is "normal," while wanting so desperately to fit in. Parents must be sensitive to the issues regarding this part of adolescence. Answer the following questions to assess how far along the ROAD to success you are.

Where Are You and Your Teen on the ROAD?

YES	NO	Check YES or NO to answer the following questions:
☐	☐	Do you avoid making negative comments about your teen's body?
☐	☐	Have you felt like you "parent" your teen less now than ever before?
☐	☐	Do you avoid pointing out your teen's flaws?
☐	☐	When your teen makes negative comments about himself or herself, do you answer with further questions instead of solutions?
☐	☐	Do you practice healthy eating?
☐	☐	Have you helped set a family schedule including mealtimes?
☐	☐	Do you and your teen eat at least five meals together each week (can include either restaurants or meals at home)?
☐	☐	Have you worked with your teen to create healthy options of meals or snacks that he or she eats independently outside of your home?
☐	☐	Have you communicated the importance of limiting screen time?
☐	☐	Do you have weekly family activities that include some form of exercise?
☐	☐	If you have a teen away from home, have you discussed healthy food options for him or her in the current living situation?
☐	☐	Do you support your teen to participate in fitness activity in or out of school?

_____ How many yes answers did you have?

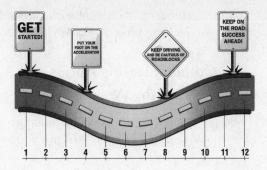

If you scored between 1 and 4, it is time to get your foot on the accelerator and focus on making small changes. If you scored between 5 and 8, you are on the ROAD to better health, but be careful of those roadblocks. If you scored between 9 and 12, use the tips in this chapter to refine and improve your goals or decisions.

The Older Teen

Teenage girls in this age group have completed most of their physical growth and development. For most girls, this occurs about four years after beginning their periods. Calorie needs of girls of this age are approaching those of adults. Teenage boys, on the other hand, experience the majority of their growth between the ages of fifteen and seventeen. Voices deepen, shoulders broaden, and growth is in full swing. Calorie needs are high, but the quality of those calories is as important. Vitamin, mineral, and protein needs increase as well.

Beyond the Physical

Along with the physical changes, other developmental milestones occur, although not on a strict schedule. In their younger days, children have concrete or black-and-white thinking. But during their teen years, they develop the ability to think abstractly. Here's an example of how that can affect weight and food choices.

Kevin is fifteen years old and is overweight by about 30 pounds. His parents have reminded him "over and over again" to stop drinking sodas. Kevin says that he has, and on further questioning reveals that he switched to lemonade.

Although Kevin "might have known better," he in fact did exactly as he was told and as a concrete thinker believed that he had accomplished the mission. As he matures, Kevin will be able to think in the abstract, such as, "If I shouldn't drink soda, then maybe all sweet drinks should become occasional treats because sweet drinks are like soda too."

Communicating About Healthy Weight

As the body and brain grow and develop, ways to communicate about food, dieting, and exercise should change as well. Tap into your teen's problem-solving skills.

Don't Tell Teens What They Already Know

Sixteen-year-old Jane is obese and also tall for her age. Her parents scheduled an appointment with a registered dietitian in hopes of helping Jane to lose some weight. While walking to the consulting room, Jane constantly tugged at her obviously tight shirt, trying to cover every piece of her body that was exposed due to the choice in clothing she'd made.

When asked what she would like to discuss during the session, Jane's mother immediately chimed in by pinching Jane's protruding abdomen and saying, "We want to lose this." Her mother proceeded to voice her disgust that Jane's shirt was "way too small." Her mother added that because Jane's father is so big, "Jane will always be a big girl."

When adolescents experience dramatic biological changes during puberty, they develop a heightened preoccupation with body image. Their increased self-awareness of the changes in their body can cause a decrease in self-esteem. For females, lower self-esteem combined with early maturation can lead to poor eating habits, like dieting and developing eating disorders. Males often experience the opposite—late maturation—which can leave them feeling inadequate and less "masculine" and lead to insecurities and self-doubt.

Noticing the physical changes in your teen is one thing, but saying them out loud is another. Don't tell your teens things they already know. Stating the obvious, especially when the focus is on your teen's body, is usually not the best way to express concern. All parents have a right to worry about their teen's weight and future health issues. But sharing that worry with your teen— especially in a negative way—may only make your teen even more self-conscious. Finding a constructive way to deal with these issues without destroying every bit of your teen's security and self-esteem is the tricky part.

Think of it from your perspective. You throw a big party for the holidays, and afterward your home is a mess. Will it help you if someone points out all the areas that need dusting and cleaning? Or let's say you make a mistake at work. How would you feel if your coworkers reminded you every day where you went wrong?

A better approach might be someone offering to help you clean your messy house, or making you feel better about the mistake by suggesting how to avoid future errors. Do the same with your teen. Instead of pointing out his or her flaws, find a way to help improve them.

The first step is to observe whether Jane perceives that her weight is a problem. If not, then the discussion should not start. Teens typically let their parents know if they think their weight is a problem. Parents who are listening to their teens will hear it.

When the teen makes a comment such as "I'm fat" or "I don't like the way I look," then you might reply. "What do you mean?" The point here is not to assume you know what she is referring to. "I don't like the way I look" may refer to skin, hair, or clothes but not weight. You won't know unless you listen and ask for more input, rather than assuming you know what the teen is thinking.

If Jane says she wants healthier food choices, then suggest you go grocery shopping together. If Jane wants to start exercising, then explore options together. Although it may take some work, it's never too late to start.

The likelihood of a dad and a son between ages fifteen and eighteen starting to practice a sport together is small if they don't have that relationship already. If the son expresses interest, go for it! If the father and son have not done things together in the past and the dad suggests it now, the teen may not warm up to the offer initially. But if the dad sticks with it, they may be able to get on track.

Set New Boundaries—for Yourself

Parents often feel scared giving up the caretaker role and watching their child become an adult. While your teen is struggling to gain his independence, you are still able to picture the day he spilled grape juice all over your new carpet. With teens, suddenly everything feels like a battle, and you are always the "bad guy."

Your life experience far outweighs what your fifteen-year-old has gone through so far, but that doesn't mean your sole purpose is to shield him from all of the struggles you wish you could have avoided in the past. As your teen moves toward his young adult years, take a step back and watch him grow and learn. You may need to bite your tongue more than once, but remember that your role is to support and guide, not live his life for him. Helping your teen make wise food choices can take restraint. Choosing food is a daily event. Constantly reminding your teen that cookies are high in calories and french fries are high in fat quickly loses its power as a helpful strategy. He will tune it out, ignore you, and go ahead and eat the foods anyway—sometimes as a declaration of independence or defiance.

▶ ROADBLOCK: Control What You Can

Try changing the home food environment without giving a lecture. Discuss your family's health and the need for everyone to eat better. Highlight healthful changes you've made in foods at home, like adding more fruits and vegetables to meals and switching from 2% to 1% milk. Alternatively, you can make the changes and not discuss why you are doing it. If your teen asks, you can say, "I need to start drinking 1% milk." Over time, the teen will either drink the 1% milk or not.

If your teen truly needs to lose weight, acknowledge his struggles by being empathetic and supportive. Support his problem-solving skills and ask how you can be of most help. Don't assume that you know what to do. Ask your teen what he needs you to do. Although it is tempting to solve the problems for your teen, sometimes the best lesson is for him to experience life himself.

Sometimes seeking outside help from a healthcare provider, such as a dietitian, can be a useful strategy. Getting guidelines and guidance from professionals helps take the pressure off of you as the parent, so you aren't in the position of being the one who is always dictating the rules. Although all parents have the wisdom of experience, sometimes it is better for your teen to hear it from someone else. Once again, approach outside support in the sense that you would like to learn as well, and that your teen is not alone in needing to find ways to improve eating and exercise habits.

Encouraging Best Behaviors

Creating a "family schedule" is like combining everyone's different activities into one long carpool route that changes daily. Suddenly you are faced with your teen bouncing from study groups, to sports practices, to school functions, to activities with friends. You may feel like asking your teen when he or she can pencil you in next. It can feel as if you've gone from being a parent to a chauffuer and eventually turning over the keys.

Save the Family Meal

Unfortunately, busy schedules can take a toll on family dynamics as well as a teen's performance in various situations. It's important to spend some time together, but it is a challenge with everyone's hectic schedules. The bigger the family, the less likely everyone is to be in the same place at the same time. Considering that we all need to eat at some point, what better time to meet than at mealtimes!

Sadly, families today are spending less time together around the kitchen table. Studies show that 22–32 percent of adolescents never or rarely (less than a few days per week) eat meals with their family. Only one-third of adolescents eat dinner with their family every day. With dinner being the most frequently consumed meal among adolescents, making this a family-oriented meal more often is important.

Another Benefit of the Family Meal

According to the National Longitudinal Study of Adolescent Health, children who ate dinner with a parent at least five days a week were more likely to get better grades and less likely to smoke or use drugs, have sex at young ages, or get into fights. Set a goal for your family to eat together more often.

A family meal not only lets a parent provide healthier choices, it also allows some time to discuss each other's lives. This family meal also serves as a "model" that your teen can mimic when away from home. Even if mealtime happens only a few times a week, it still is a special time together. One word of warning: Keep conversations at the table away from food and dieting; focus more on talking about the day's events, current events, upcoming school activities, and so on.

This family meal doesn't have to be elaborate or time-consuming to prepare. Instead of traditional fast food, think fast and easy. Consider tuna salad sandwiches made with low-fat mayo on whole wheat toast, "bag salad" with low-fat dressing, and precut fruit. Add some pretzels or a baked potato with just a touch of margarine and you have a meal in fifteen minutes or less. Fast does not mean a drive-through restaurant.

Independent Food Choices

As your teen becomes a young adult, she will make more and more food choices without your supervision. Research shows that 25–50 percent of a teen's meals are eaten away from home. Help your teen find ways to choose wisely when facing a fast-food menu and other nutritional dilemmas.

Angela and her mother both want to eat healthy foods without cutting out all of their favorites including "anything involving a fast-food window." Angela consistently stops at these restaurants with friends, and because her mother has "given up on cooking," she finds herself taking the "easy way out" on most nights as well.

Instead of pointing the finger at each other about who instilled these habits and who is at fault for giving in to temptations, both mother and daughter agree that they are each to blame. Angela says that she "knows there are healthier options to choose" and that she needs to "stop giving in to the smell of fries." Her mother says that she would like to try to have more meals at home, making it "easier to stay away from the not so healthy fast-food choices." Both agree that it would be fun to start cooking together at home; they consider the idea of taking a cooking class together.

They decide that if their only option requires a fast-food night, they are going to look for healthier options, such as a side salad instead of fries or a grilled chicken sandwich instead of nuggets. Of course, they will probably include fries at some time during the week, but it "will no longer be an every night side dish or an after-school snack."

Angela and her mother found a great way to resolve an issue together. Assigning blame never results in productive learning, while working together for resolutions makes change so much easier. Learning is an ongoing process. Even the most aware parent can learn something new.

Seek information from the appropriate healthcare providers or reliable sources of nutrition information. Work together with your family to make the necessary changes in your family. As you travel down the ROAD, think about some of the important decisions you will have to consider with your teen. Some of the issues you may face include dining out, dating, and liquid calories.

Eating Out

During adolescence, teens begin to spend less time with the family and more time with their peers. This means meals are going to consist of more school food and fast food, and fewer hearty cooked meals at home. Teens who normally eat a balanced meal of meat, potatoes, and some vegetables at home more often than not change to a bag of chips and a soda at school or with friends, hardly a well-balanced meal.

Where Do Teens Get Their Meals?

Teens eat one-third of their meals away from home. Where?

School	52%
Fast food	16%

| Other locations | 26% |
| Vending machines | 6% |

Finding the proper nutritional balance can be tricky, but better choices are available in almost every eating situation away from home. In a vending machine, for example, baked chips or pretzels and a diet soda (or better yet, water) make an okay snack. When possible, throw in a piece of fruit to increase the nutrition content and make it more filling.

Most fast-food restaurants have healthier options so you are less restricted to that same old grilled chicken sandwich with nothing on it. Choose a side salad with a light dressing instead of fries, never super-size anything, and choose the smaller sandwich instead of the larger one.

▶ **ROADBLOCK: Do Small Changes *Really* Make a Difference?**
Making little changes can make a big difference in caloric intake. For example, choosing a chicken fajita pita, side salad with light dressing, piece of fruit, and a diet cola versus a sourdough cheeseburger, seasoned curly fries, and a regular cola saves you up to 900 calories—an entire meal allotment for most people! The rule of thumb in most restaurants is:

- Go for the smallest portions or split an entrée.
- Choose the grilled or baked items versus the fried.
- Most important, fill up on fruits and vegetables.

Making It Multicultural

If you like foreign food, become more familiar with the language that signals higher-fat choices. Be sure to ask the waiter for details on what's in a sauce or dressing if you don't know. For specific tips on better choices when trying different cuisines, go back to the restaurant lists in Chapter 3.

Group Functions or Dating: Keep It Lite

Most parents, especially those with daughters, dread the time when the teen proposes the idea of dating. But dating at this age isn't always what it used to be. Although teens do date one-on-one, they more often go out in groups. When not on a date, they may be together at study groups or sports and school functions.

When going out on a date or with a group of friends, most social events revolve around food. Even if food isn't the primary objective, there's candy, soda, and popcorn at the movies or pizza or a snack bar at the bowling alley. Some teens may find it embarrassing or boring to be the one who makes healthier choices in a social situation. Help them find ways to respond to any comments about their healthy choices. For example, they can say, "I'm eating smart now because I'm going to live to be 102." Or if they play sports, they might say, "I'm learning how to improve my performance through the things I eat."

If friends are teasing her for trying to take care of her body, then maybe those friends aren't the best ones for her. Typically, people look for friends with common interests, which is especially important when dating. A great bond for friends can be working toward a goal of being healthier together.

If your teen maintains healthy eating habits throughout the week, then enjoying an occasional treat out with friends can be okay. Depending on the choices she made throughout the week, if your teen finds herself on a dining date, she can use her nutrition knowledge to make balanced choices.

Another tactic you can suggest is to take advantage of being a twosome and split a meal. In most restaurants, an entrée easily adds up to almost a day's worth of calories. For most people, stopping at the halfway mark is hard when an enticing food is in front of them. Planning ahead to split a meal is always the best option—and your teen can put the money she saves toward a treat without calories.

Liquid Calories

Ben is fifteen years old and has been told he is obese. Ben's dad can't understand how someone who is "so active" could fall into the obese category. When asked the kinds of activities performed, Ben says he plays baseball, with practices four nights and one game every week. Practice consists of a number of drills, some weight training, and some light jogging. Ben's dad comments that Ben eats less than his teammates but usually chooses "all-natural drinks such as lemonade and fruit punch." Ben also consumes two 32-ounce bottles of sports drink every day. And that's the problem.

Liquid calories can be dangerous. They don't fill you up because they don't last long in the stomach, yet they usually contribute extra calories on top of those consumed through food. Commercials about sports and energy drinks are everywhere, falsely showing that they lead to a healthy, sleek physique.

No doubt these drinks serve a useful purpose for endurance athletes who need hydration and electrolyte replenishment, and provide improvement for exercise or sports that last more than one hour. But they are not for routine fluid intake and not necessary for exercise that lasts less than an hour. For that purpose water works just fine.

"All-natural" doesn't mean that the calories are low, either. Adding up just the liquid calories, Ben consumed over 800 calories. Controlling the liquid calories is the key to controlling Ben's weight.

Calories from the Unthinkable

Most parents don't want to imagine that their sixteen-year-old would ever think about drinking a drop of alcohol. But the truth of the matter is that peer pressure gets the best of all of us, and many kids are consuming alcoholic beverages at young ages. Regardless of age, alcohol can be a big hindrance to weight loss.

Alcohol contains 7 calories per gram. Calorie intake can range anywhere from 100 calories in a light beer up to 400 calories in drinks combining alcohol with a sugar-loaded juice or soda. These empty calories easily add up. Because of peer pressure, and lack of judgment caused by the effects of alcohol, many do not stop at just one drink.

According to the federal government's 2005 Dietary Guidelines for Americans, moderate drinking is defined as up to one drink per day for women and two drinks per day for men. That does not mean having seven drinks on a weekend because you abstained all week—a common habit among younger drinkers. Because alcoholic drinks contain a lot of calories, this is obviously a major roadblock to any weight-loss program. For adults, this does not necessarily mean cutting out alcohol altogether: As with everything, moderation is key. The bottom line for alcohol consumption in the adolescent age group, aside from the fact that it is illegal, is that it makes weight loss difficult.

Heading Off to College or Work

Heading off to college or entering the workforce is an exciting time in life, but such an enormous transition is also stressful. A common concern for any high school student is the mysterious weight gain everyone acquires when entering the real world. So where do these dreaded 15 pounds come from?

> *Jackie is heading off to college in the fall. She is excited but very anxious about the unknown. When asked what she will study, she is not sure yet. When asked what she is looking forward to most, she is once again unsure but talks about the independence of "living on my own without parents telling me what to do."*
>
> *When asked what she is most nervous about, she is quick to answer: "The freshman fifteen, of course!"*

One of the big challenges of heading to college or the work world is learning how to adjust to the newly gained independence, including meal choices.

Teens who are used to having most of their food provided for them must choose every single meal on their own. Whether shopping themselves at the grocery store or living in a dorm with the convenience of a cafeteria, they still must decide which choices are best while facing a daily supply of french fries and ice cream.

Students also start pulling their first all-nighters, leaving them exhausted with little or no energy for extra activity. The constant social gatherings filled with tempting foods, alcoholic beverages, and energy drinks also cause kids to pack on the calories—inevitably leading to that extra 15 pounds. But there are ways to handle these challenges.

Following are some tips you can offer your teen (adults can follow them too).

Dorm Food

As with any restaurant, go into a dorm or college cafeteria knowing the healthier choices to aim for.

- Know your portion sizes, especially for buffet-style cafeterias.
- Look for the salad bar and fill at least half of your plate.
- Pay attention to low-fat options, such as low-fat dairy (milk or yogurt), lean meat (grilled or baked chicken, fish, turkey, etc.), and low-fat dressings.
- Don't completely deprive yourself of french fries and sweets, but eat them in moderation. Do your best to fill up on the other food group items first.

Work

In a work setting you may find yourself dining out more often or constantly surrounded by treats in the break room. Follow these suggestions for helping with self-control:

- Avoid dining out every day of the week by bringing your own lunch—a great way to limit calories and make the right choices.
- When going out to lunch with friends, find the healthier choices on the menu (see the dining out tips starting on page 65).
- In the break room, steer clear of the snacks when you are really hungry.
- Keep your own healthy snack options on hand to make it easier to avoid temptation.
- Do enjoy some treats every now and then—just don't eat them on an empty stomach (when it's harder to stay within reason about your portion sizes).

- Never set yourself up for failure by having a huge bowl filled with your favorite tempting treats right on your desk. The calories in miniature candy bars add up quickly. Fill the bowl with something less tempting, like mints, if you feel the need to put anything there at all.

Social Gatherings

Attending social gatherings when you are trying to lose or maintain weight can be hard. Finger foods are everywhere, and although they don't seem like they have a huge amount of calories, they can really add up. Consuming a large amount of calories without knowing how many also happens when you're preoccupied by your surroundings.

- Be conscious of what you eat by placing everything on a plate before eating anything.
- Hold a drink in your dominant hand, so you are less able to unconsciously grab food items as you pass.
- If there is a vegetable or fruit tray, fill up on that first.
- Make your own low-fat dishes to bring along—your hostess will appreciate it and so will others who are more health conscious like you.
- Eat defensively by having a low-calorie snack, such as low-fat popcorn, before you go to a party or study break where they're serving pizza.

Physical Activity

By the time the average person reaches the age of seventy, he or she has spent the equivalent of seven to ten years watching TV. Meanwhile, the lack of physical activity is one of the main causes of obesity, contributing to at least three hundred thousand preventable deaths per year.

Losing Out on Sports and Physical Education

Even with statistics showing that people need more exercise, physical education in schools has greatly declined. High schoolers just aren't getting enough exercise. The 2003 Youth Risk Behavior Survey shows:

- Nationwide, only 28.4 percent of high school students attend a physical education class five days per week.
- Nationwide, 11.5 percent of students had not participated in either

vigorous physical activity or moderate physical activity during the seven days preceding the survey.

- Overall, the prevalence of no vigorous or moderate physical activity was higher among eleventh (13.7 percent) and twelfth graders (14.0 percent) than ninth graders (9.1 percent).
- Nationwide, 57.6 percent of students had played on one or more sports teams during the twelve months preceding the survey, and this was higher among males than females.

Girls' Decreasing Activity

Adolescence is the time when girls in particular are much less likely to exercise or play sports. One theory is that girls become more concerned about makeup and hair and don't want exercise to mess it up or to take time to fix after exercise. It is also possible that girls this age don't want to sweat or get dirty.

The Youth Risk Behavior Survey shows that:

- 22.1 percent of girls participated in regular activity compared to 28.9 percent of boys.
- 51 percent of girls participated on sports teams compared to 64 percent of boys.

With so much focus on body image at this age, exercise is more important than ever. To maintain healthy growth patterns, adolescent girls need to participate in some type of physical activity.

The 1996 Surgeon General's Report, *Physical Activity and Health,* discusses the many benefits of physical activity—including reduced stress and anxiety, as well as increased self-esteem. Physical activity has been shown to improve the ability to sleep, increase attentiveness, and raise energy levels. According to the American College of Sports Medicine, those who participate in sports at an early age are more likely to remain active in their adult years. Therefore, encouraging children to participate in activities during early childhood and adolescence can possibly produce great results for improved health in the general population.

Exercise as a Personal Choice

Michael is fifteen years old and overweight. He used to be very active, but recently he does not have any time and hates to exercise. On a visit to his doctor to "lose weight," he is asked if he used to enjoy any kind of activities.

Michael says that his mom used to "make me walk on the treadmill every night for 30 minutes." Michael also states that he just got a new computer game at home and would "play it all day" if he didn't have school.

For many people, the most difficult part of exercise is actually finding time to do it. Studies show that adolescents watch up to 3 or more hours of TV a day, but if you ask them to perform 20–30 minutes of exercise, it's like you're asking them to climb Mt. Everest. The key is to find something you actually enjoy. The problem is that when most people hear the word *exercise,* they envision themselves on a treadmill seven days a week—marching along at the same speed for the same amount of time. Even for fitness experts that regime sounds miserable!

Before trying to force your teen to join a gym, think back to your teen years when moving was actually fun because it meant recess or playing with your friends. Was your best memory at the roller rink? Take up Rollerblading. Did you love the summertime because it meant daily visits to the pool? Join a swim team. Was your favorite game tag or chase? Perfect for the jogger in all of us. Do you find yourself tapping to the beat every time your favorite song comes on the radio? A dance class or video may be perfect for you.

Exercise is not about which machine you are going to strap yourself to for an hour each day. Exercise is more about moving your body and burning those calories. And just like your favorite TV show that you reserve time for, if you love the activity you've chosen, you're more likely to make the time to do it.

So how much time should you make for exercise and activity? Being active throughout the day is important. Whether you're a student or a full-time worker, think of the time you spend at a desk or computer—and watching TV when you get home. Adding up those hours throughout the week can show why extra calories add up and increase weight gain.

Becoming more conscious of sitting time versus moving time is crucial. In addition to getting aerobic activity, make sure you do little things throughout your day to increase movement. For example, take the stairs instead of the elevator, perform housework or yard work, and walk around (or even stand) while talking on the phone. Even walking through the shopping mall is considered exercise!

Just as making little changes to the calories you consume can make a big difference over time, so can making little changes to the calories you use. This example shows the estimated calories a 150-pound person burns in one day:

Sit or Be Fit

ACTIVITY PERFORMED	CALORIES BURNED
Sitting on the couch (30 minutes)	40
Standing while talking on phone (30 minutes)	60
Performing household chores (30 minutes)	85
Walking around mall (30 minutes)	150
Riding bike to and from school (30 minutes total—15 minutes each way)	270
Swimming laps at low intensity (30 minutes)	260

Compared to spending your free time outside of school or work on the couch or in front of a computer, you reap quite a benefit just from just keeping yourself moving!

Since the 1996 Surgeon General's Report on Physical Activity and Health, it was recommended that all adolescents be physically active most days of the week, whether that includes play, games, sports, work, transportation, recreation, or physical education. The Dietary Guidelines 2005 recently updated these recommendations, again stating that children and adolescents have 60 minutes of moderate to vigorous physical activity (causing them to sweat and breathe hard) daily or on most days of the week. This does not need to be at one time; it can be cumulative throughout the day. These moderate to vigorous activities can include walking, jogging, biking, light to heavy yard work, dancing, and more.

Cheering On Your Teen

Although adolescents are highly influenced by their peers, family also plays an important role in encouraging them to stay active. A child at this age is more likely to participate in sports or other activities if parents or siblings do too.

The Smith family came in with the focus on their fifteen-year-old daughter Laura, who is overweight and very inactive. Both parents are also overweight and neither exercises regularly. When discussing possible options to increase daily activity, Laura made it very clear that she cannot drive but was willing to go to the gym where some of her friends go if someone would just take her.

According to the American College of Sports Medicine, if both parents are physically active, the teen is six times more likely to be physically active. Once again, parents are the role models.

Another of your responsibilities is to support your teen in his or her chosen activities and provide access or transportation to convenient play spaces or recreation centers. Finding ways to participate in their sports, whether it is attending a game or practice, assisting in drill work outside of practice, or taking the time to ask questions to get more familiar with their sport, encourages your teen's continued participation.

Not only are you the parent, now you have become top cheerleader. Studies prove that those who participate in sports at an early age most likely perform better in school due to an increase in alertness and also have greater success in becoming more physically active at a later age. Showing your positive support from the sidelines increases the likelihood that your teen will want to continue to build on his or her talents.

It is great to support your child, but watch out for the fine line between being a positive cheerleader and being that obnoxious parent who is living vicariously through his or her teen. The American College of Sports Medicine categorized the various parents seen in youth sports:

- Mr. and Mrs. Agenda, who overschedule their teen
- Mr. and Mrs. Braggadocio, who constantly gloat about their teen's supposed successes
- Mr. and Mrs. Hothead, who start to behave inappropriately the minute the game begins
- Mr. and Mrs. Over-Indulgence, who reward to excess and/or shower their teen with top-of-the-line apparel

Sometimes a little too much support can result in too much pressure that can lead to "burnout" or a dislike for any sport or activity in the future. Various eating disorders can stem from the overbearing parent or coach, while also damaging the teen's original enjoyment.

Sometimes with or without parents' added pressures, adolescents involved in sports push themselves beyond their limits. Overtraining can create both physical and psychological effects. When an athlete becomes unenthusiastic about the sport or acquires repeated injuries, parents should consider whether overtraining may be a factor. Parents, coaches, and teachers are responsible for being aware of a young athlete's needs and should respond to any signs that suggest a teen's enjoyment of a sport is waning.

Seeking Advice

During adolescence, it is not uncommon for your teen to seek out the advice of others in order to lose weight. Peers, popular magazines, and the Internet are instant sources of medical and weight-loss advice. Some of it is good, but some is downright dangerous. If needed, seek the help of a qualified professional or team of professionals. Your teen's primary care provider may have expertise in practical dietary counseling. However, a registered dietitian is needed whenever moving past the basic recommendations.

Some physicians work well with teens; others don't. Look for a physician who is comfortable listening to and talking with teens. If you see behavioral barriers to implementing weight loss, consider consulting a mental-health provider. An exercise professional may be indicated in some cases, but basic exercises such as walking, running, swimming, and playing do not require an expert.

Setting Goals for Your Teen

Whatever goals your family sets for food and exercise, at this stage your teen must be making decisions on his own with a little guidance from Mom and Dad. Allow your teen to set reasonable goals for exercise and nutrition. Sample goals he may consider:

- Increasing physical activity with friends to three times per week
- Controlling liquid calories and choosing healthier options at least once per week when eating out with friends
- Parking farther from the store entrance anywhere he goes this week

Fiction: I wasn't a chubby kid in my early years at school, so I'm not going to be obese when I'm older.

Fact: More teenagers are obese than any other children's age group, which shows that weight "catches up" with kids as they get older. Research shows a pattern that makes this a particular problem for African-American children, who often remain thin until they approach adolescence and then gain a lot of weight in a short time.

PART III

• • •

Considering the Next Steps

10

. . .

When Your Child
Needs an Expert

Overweight/morbid obesity is no longer a disease limited to adults; it is now the most common nutritional disorder of children and adolescents in the United States. The number of children who are severely overweight has almost doubled in the past twenty years.

Obesity is a critical issue because it can lead or add to the development of numerous potentially life-threatening diseases referred to as *comorbidities,* and these diseases also are on the rise. Comorbidities can take years off your life. A study by Kevin Fontaine and colleagues followed obese adolescents for thirty years and showed that they have more chronic disease and die earlier than adults who were normal weight as adolescents. The obesity epidemic has multiple causes:

- Calorie-dense processed foods are plentiful.
- Portions are larger.
- Physical education requirements in schools have decreased.
- Some parents have fears of letting their children outside to play.
- Our perception of a normal-sized child has changed.
- We are bombarded with commercial messages urging us to eat more food—and make it fast food and super-size portions.

Let's not forget nutritional misinformation: high fat, low fat, high protein, no carbs, low carbs, good carbs, bad carbs, glycemic load, eating only raw foods, sugar portrayed as the "anti-nutrient," eating foods defined by our blood type, and the list goes on.

Meanwhile, our lifestyles are more sedentary than our ancestors' and labor-saving devices keep us from being active. The human body was designed to store fat as a survival mechanism so that our ancestors wouldn't starve when they couldn't find food. It was not designed to overeat high-fat processed foods and then sit in front of a computer or TV screen for the greater part of the day.

Earlier chapters highlighted some simple steps to follow to prevent and manage overweight. Your child may need an expert if you have tried many of the tips throughout this book without success or if you have been told that your child is above the 95th percentile BMI or diagnosed as obese. Aggressive approaches may be indicated if you have been told your child has a health condition associated with being overweight or comorbidity.

Clearly a BMI of greater than the 95th percentile for age increases your child's likelihood of having a health risk associated with excess weight. Although excess weight tends to run in families, as BMI increases, so does the risk of health consequences. Sometimes overweight is hard to see; that is why the measurement of BMI is crucial. Check your child's BMI using the formula in Appendix B (it explains how to use the table below) and take a good look at your action plan. It may be time to get out the big guns!

BMI COMPARISON BETWEEN ADULTS AND CHILDREN

Adults		Children Ages 2–20 (percentile for age)
< 18.5	Underweight	
18.5–24.9	Normal weight	< 5th Underweight
25–29.9	Overweight	85th–< 95th Overweight
30–40	Obese	
> 40	Extremely obese	≥ 95th Obese

The treatment of adolescent obesity involves more than a simple attempt to eat less, follow a fad diet, or take diet pills. Because young people's bodies and brains are still developing, their responses can be hard to predict and possibly dangerous. Also, effective weight loss typically comes from an organized plan and solid support from a knowledgeable team.

If your child is overweight, ask your pediatrician or healthcare provider to help you to assemble a weight-loss team. Keep in mind that the most important members of the team are your child and your family. Building lasting change begins in the family: healthcare providers just supply the tools.

Your Medical Weight-Loss Team

There are at least six players:

- *Physician.* Find a physician who specializes in pediatric or adolescent medicine. Pediatricians and adolescent specialists are in tune with the unique needs of teens—especially important since most Americans cite their doctor as their main source of health information. The physician's role is to evaluate the child to rule out medical causes for the obesity and to assess and monitor any risk factors secondary to the obesity. The physician may order blood work periodically to keep track of medical improvement.

- *Registered dietitian.* Look for the R.D. (registered dietitian) credential to make sure you are receiving the best nutritional care for your teen. You can locate an R.D. in your area through the American Dietetic Association (www.eatright.org). A nutritionist is not the same as an R.D. "Nutritionist" is not a legally protected title, so anyone can call himself or herself one. The R.D. credentials are based on extensive training in specialized areas of expertise. The dietitian works with the medical team and advises them on the best weight-loss strategy to try. In addition, the dietitian works with the family on selecting healthy foods, understanding food groups, and determining appropriate food qualities and portion sizes. He or she also provides help with grocery shopping, food preparation, and making good choices when eating out. Dietitians can also help to identify roadblocks and solutions.

- *Exercise professional.* Physical therapists or exercise physiologists are experts in designing programs to improve fitness, especially if a child is limited by health concerns. Studies also suggest that a personal trainer can improve adherence to an exercise program and enhance weight-loss outcomes. Exercise alone is rarely enough to promote weight loss. However, the National Weight Control Registry indicates that people who exercise most often are most successful at keeping weight off. The exercise professional determines the child's fitness level and incorporates an appropriate exercise routine into the child's lifestyle. In some settings the exercise professional may supervise the exercise program. In sessions with an exercise professional, families learn about different types of exercise goals. The exercise professional also helps to motivate families to stick to their exercise programs.

- *Mental-health professional.* A mental-health professional such as a trained psychologist is a must on a weight-loss team. Studies show that overweight children are often depressed, which may be a barrier to successful weight loss. Choose a psychologist who has experience and enjoys working with children. The issues facing especially teens can be daunting, and a trained therapist can help your child navigate the challenges of weight loss. The psychologist is responsible for assessing the family and child in regard to the appropriateness of beginning a weight-loss program. The psychologist looks specifically at how ready the family is for change and what family support is available to the child, who will be asked to make major changes in behavior.

- *Parents*. Family is a crucial part of every child's weight-loss team. Stay involved!
- *Child*. Finally, but most important, your child must be enthusiastic about the plan and the team members.

Changing Behavior

Because weight control for children can be influenced by many factors, including emotions, home environment, media, and friends, it is crucial that a weight-management program address all these aspects. A program that takes a cognitive behavioral, multidisciplinary approach is best to fulfill this need.

Cognitive behavioral therapy emphasizes that thoughts and feelings often dictate our actions. For example, if you feel bored, there is a thought that snacking will make you feel better. This thought leads to the action of overeating. Cognitive behavioral therapists teach ways to deal with unwanted thoughts and feelings, and the behaviors that follow, by identifying what is the root cause. After the cause is identified, new ways of thinking and feeling are learned, and replaced by thoughts that lead to more desirable actions.

All members of the weight-loss team are responsible for implementing the program with the child and family. The team establishes a supportive relationship with the child and the parents. They teach the techniques in the program and help the family apply them. The mental-health professional may also assess for barriers, such as depression, bullying, or teasing, and their effects on the child.

From the beginning, the emphasis of any weight-management program should be on changes in lifestyle rather than simply changes in weight. Cognitive behavioral therapy can lead to lasting changes in the child's behavior. A weight-management program will incorporate many different cognitive behavioral techniques. One of the essential techniques taught should be self-monitoring, which is often done in the form of a food and exercise journal. Self-monitoring will help the child and family to understand "patterns" in eating and exercise so that those patterns leading to excessive weight gain can eventually be changed. Typical self-monitored items are amount of food, kind of food, time of meals, who you were with when you ate your meal, what you were doing, and how you were feeling. The idea is that behavior must be monitored before the child can make changes.

Other behavior modification techniques that should be incorporated in a weight-management program are recognizing behavior chains or patterns. Helping the child become more aware of these eating patterns will help her understand where she can begin to take control and make changes. A child can begin to develop a list of fun activities and also a "need-to-do" list that she can use to substitute for unwanted eating behaviors. Remind her that items on the list must be activities that she really will do. Parents may need to help the child negotiate for greater opportunities.

No Magic Wand

Every year Americans spend tens of billions of dollars on weight-loss products and services. Most plans work initially but fail to provide lasting results. Many popular diets recommend limiting single nutrients or entire food groups. Although they may bring modest weight loss, you may not be improving your overall health by omitting grains or fruits and vegetables, which are essential to a healthier lifestyle (when accompanied by daily activity).

When considering a diet or weight-loss program, avoid plans that promise a quick fix, require you to stop eating certain foods or food groups, rely on testimonials as "evidence," and sound too good to be true.

Fad diets typically promote quick results, but most of them are too rigid, making long-term compliance difficult. Some can make you lose weight quickly, but watch out! When you fail to continue with such diets and return to previous eating habits, the weight comes back just as quickly, and you may even gain back more pounds than you lost.

Excess weight is not gained overnight, so it won't go away overnight. It takes time and effort.

Lost Time

Monitoring your weight is also important statistically in terms of life expectancy. Being morbidly obese (BMI ≥ 45) at twenty years of age results in a loss of life expectancy of:

- 22 years for African-American males
- 12 years for white males
- 8 years for white females
- 4 years for African-American females

Keeping Weight Off

Research from the National Weight Control Registry shows that people who are successful at losing weight and keeping it off do the following:

- monitor and record food choices
- eat a low-fat diet with a reduction in sugars
- participate in regular moderate exercise
- eat breakfast
- eat a consistent diet from day to day

Losing weight and keeping it off is a challenge, but the benefits are great. Clearly, reducing calorie intake and increasing exercise remain the key ingredients to any successful plan. A quick fix, however, is not a lasting solution. The weight-loss industry makes billions of dollars on the promise of the latest and greatest diet, pill, or potion for weight loss. These are not healthy. More important, they aren't effective in the long-term. Medical options often include a more rigorous approach for weight control in an attempt to reduce the co-morbidities associated with excess weight.

Very Low-Calorie Diet (VLCD)

By definition, very low-calorie diets contain fewer than 800 calories per day. They may be a liquid diet or made up of limited amounts of regular foods. In certain situations, highly specialized diets may be prescribed by a physician or registered dietitian to induce rapid weight loss.

These diets typically are very low in carbohydrates such as grains, fruits, vegetables, and fats. One particular type of VLCD is the protein-sparing modified fast. Although on the surface it appears to be the same as many of the low-carbohydrate diets of recent years, there are some important differences.

The popular versions suggest that calories don't count and that counting carbohydrates is all that matters. Nothing is farther from the truth. Paying attention to calories is always important. The protein-sparing modified fast also limits the amount of animal fat by focusing only on lean meats. This diet promotes rapid weight loss by forcing the body to use its own fat for energy, a process called ketosis. Large amounts of fluid are lost, causing a rapid decrease in weight. Because this diet is very low in calories, it is referred to as a "modified fast." Because the diet is so restrictive, patients are at risk for developing vitamin and mineral deficiencies, which can be detrimental to their long-term health; prescribed supplements are needed.

Medical professionals do not recommend these sorts of diets without ongoing supervision. They are very restrictive, difficult to sustain, and likely to cause side effects. As with most diets, and particularly those that are very restrictive, noncompliance (failure to stick to their rules) is an issue. However, if your child has a BMI of greater than 30 or has failed at traditional weight loss, this type of medically supervised diet may be the motivation needed to "jump-start" the weight-loss process. It is not designed as a long-term solution.

> ▶ HELPFUL HINT: **Keep It Safe and Avoid Health Fraud**
> Diet and physical activity are keys to weight loss, and there is always the temptation to find an alternative to make the process easier and quicker. Many of the so-called natural supplements marketed for weight loss may not be as safe as they claim. Unlike prescription medicines, the FDA does not test dietary or herbal supplements for purity or effectiveness before they reach the market. According to the FDA red flags for fraud include:
>
> * one product does it all
> * personal testimonials instead of science
> * promises of a quick fix and easy weight loss
> * the use of the term *all-natural*
> * new scientific breakthrough
> * satisfaction guaranteed
> * paranoid accusations against mainstream healthcare
> * meaningless medical jargon

Although supplements claim to be safe, science suggests there are risks involved. Ephedra, a weight-loss herb, was banned by the FDA in 2004 after deaths were associated with this product. Currently, two types of natural weight-loss supplements are on the market. Synephrine, ephedra's cousin, marketed as bitter orange or Citrus aurantium, has been implicated in cases of stroke and ischemic colitis. Green tea extract as a supplement increases the likelihood of liver disease. "All-natural" does not equal safe or effective.

The Health Consequences of Too Much Weight

If your child is obese, he or she has significant health risks called *comorbidities*. Children and adolescents above the 95th percentile for BMI are significantly more likely to remain overweight as adults and suffer health consequences of obesity. These include:

* excess insulin
* metabolic syndrome
* Type 2 diabetes
* heart disease
* liver disease

- obstructive sleep apnea
- orthopedic problems
- pseudotumor cerebri
- depression

All of these comorbid conditions have the potential to be reversed with weight loss, physical activity, and healthier eating habits.

Our bodies give us warning signs that problems are on the way. It is important to recognize the early warning signs. As excess weight increases, the body makes an attempt to keep everything on the "inside" working well, but it becomes harder to do with increasing weight. One of the problems associated with excess weight is an increase in insulin production.

Insulin

Insulin is a building hormone. Its job is to take glucose out of the blood and deliver it to the cells inside the body to make fuel or store it. The problem with an excess amount of insulin is that it makes it harder to lose weight, which is a catabolic or breaking-down process. Excess insulin can contribute to many of the comorbidities of overweight. As weight increases, resistance to insulin can occur, and the body makes more insulin to compensate. As a building hormone, insulin can cause excess pigment to be deposited in the creases of the skin. This is called acanthosis nigricans.

Acanthosis Nigricans

Acanthosis nigricans is the outward sign that your child is developing insulin resistance. It is a dark velvety pigment that develops in the creases of the skin, most notably around the neck. Excess insulin stimulates the body to produce more pigment or color in the skin. It often is mistaken for poor hygiene and adolescents attempt to scrub it off.

What Is Hyperinsulinemia?

Insulin is a vital hormone made by the pancreas. It helps to take glucose and other nutrients out of the blood and delivers nutrition to muscles, organs, and tissues. With increasing weight, the pancreas works harder to keep up with the demand. At the same time the pancreas is making more insulin, the body becomes resistant to the insulin, signaling a further demand on the pancreas to produce more and more insulin. This insulin resistance is thought to contribute to heart disease, high blood pressure, and some forms of cancer.

Metabolic Syndrome

Metabolic syndrome, also called insulin resistance syndrome, is a group of symptoms that increases the chances of developing Type 2 diabetes and heart disease. The risk of metabolic syndrome can be seen both on the outside and on the inside. On the outside, where you store your fat, your physical shape can help you to decide if you are at increased risk.

▶ HELPFUL HINT: **Apple or Pear?**
An apple body type is one where the majority of the excess weight is seen above the belly button. Excess weight in the abdomen and upper back are the usual location. For adult women, a waist measurement greater than 35 inches is the red flag of belly fat. For men, it is a circumference of greater than 40 inches. Research is ongoing to develop standards for children and teens.
A pear-shaped body means most of the fat is located below the belly button. Having a pear-shaped body reduces the risk of metabolic syndrome.

Hormone changes on the inside of the body can cause acanthosis nigricans to appear, usually on the back of the neck. Any of these three symptoms indicates metabolic syndrome:

* Excessive fat stored in and around the abdomen giving the appearance of an apple-shaped body
* Insulin resistance or elevated blood sugar
* High levels of triglycerides, a blood fat
* Low levels of HDL, the good cholesterol
* High blood pressure

In the Third National Health and Nutrition Examination Survey (NHANES III) metabolic syndrome was diagnosed in one out of three overweight or obese adolescents using the National Cholesterol Education Program Guidelines. Additionally, two out of three adolescents showed at least one of the criteria.

Type 2 Diabetes

In a nutshell, diabetes is an imbalance between insulin production or utilization and glucose uptake by the cells. As childhood obesity has increased, so has the incidence of Type 2 diabetes in adolescents and youth. It is estimated that for children born in the year 2000, there is a one in three chance of developing this disease. In the past, Type 2 diabetes was commonly referred to as "adult onset" and Type 1 diabetes as "juvenile onset." This is no longer the case, as more and more children are being diagnosed with Type 2 diabetes.

Signs and symptoms of diabetes are subtle and increase in severity over time. Common signs and symptoms are:

- fatigue
- excessive thirst
- excessive urination
- excessive hunger
- slow healing of sores
- difficulty concentrating
- acanthosis nigricans (dark pigmentation of the skin)
- metabolic syndrome

There are several alterations to this metabolic process that are related to childhood obesity. One is insulin resistance, or what is commonly referred to as prediabetes. Here, the pancreas is producing insulin, but the body is not recognizing it. Even though there is plenty of insulin in the blood, the sugar cannot get into the cells. Cells throughout the body become less sensitive to insulin and the pancreas compensates by producing more insulin. Over time, the pancreas cannot keep up with the demand and blood sugar levels start to rise.

Insulin also helps the body store excess calories in the fat cells. Therefore, people with insulin resistance have an increased tendency to store fat and gain weight. Weight gain can in turn change the body chemistry, thus causing further weight gain. Over time, the insulin-producing cells of the pancreas can no longer sustain the high insulin production rate and die off. These cells may also be damaged by excess fat deposits within the pancreas itself, causing a rise in blood sugar levels.

Type 2 diabetes occurs more in African Americans, Hispanics, American Indians, and Asians. Other risk factors for developing Type 2 diabetes are family history of Type 2 diabetes, low birth weight, maternal diabetes, overweight or obesity, and puberty. During puberty the body becomes more resistant to insulin, which is a risk factor for development of Type 2 diabetes, particularly in an overweight child.

Screening for Diabetes

The American Diabetes Association and the American Academy of Pediatrics recommend screening for Type 2 diabetes for children over the age of ten, or at the onset of puberty if it occurs before the age of ten, who are overweight (BMI above 85th percentile, or weight for height greater than 85th percentile, or weight greater than 120 percent ideal) and have two of the following additional risk factors:

- Family history of Type 2 diabetes in first- or second-degree relative (first degree: parent, sibling, child; second degree: grandparent, aunt, or uncle)
- race/ethnicity: African American, American Indian, Asian, Hispanic/Latino, or Pacific Islander
- signs of insulin resistance or conditions associated with insulin resistance: acanthosis nigricans, hypertension, dyslipidemia (disruption of lipids—fats—in the blood), or polycystic ovary syndrome

Type 2 diabetes is a very serious, lifelong disease. Controlling blood sugar levels is the key to leading a healthy life. The recommendations presented in this chapter are only an overview. Consult with your healthcare provider for the best plan to manage your child's diabetes.

Heart Disease

Obese children are at risk for heart disease (also called *cardiovascular disease*). Studies reveal that some precursors to heart disease start in adolescence. Development of atherosclerosis (narrowing of the arteries by cholesterol and other substances) can begin in early childhood and develop over decades. Heart-related risk factors that are common in obese children include:

- Elevated blood lipids. Low HDL (good) cholesterol and elevated triglycerides, LDL (bad) cholesterol, or total cholesterol.
- Elevated body mass index.
- Elevated blood pressure. The heart must work harder to pump blood to the body, which can lead to other conditions such as stroke, kidney failure, heart failure, heart attack, and vision problems.
- Sleep apnea: Characterized by excessive snoring where breathing stops repeatedly. This interrupted sleep can cause abnormal blood clotting.

Nonalcoholic Fatty Liver Disease

Nonalcoholic fatty liver disease describes a range of conditions, from the mildest—accumulation of fat within the liver—to nonalcoholic steatohepatitis (NASH), which is potentially serious. NASH is associated with inflammation and scarring of the liver that may eventually lead to cirrhosis, a long-term disease that can develop into irreversible scarring and possibly liver failure.

How Does the Liver Get Sick?

The liver is an amazing organ. It is the largest internal organ in the body, one of the most essential, and it's the only one that has the power to regenerate itself. That means that if the liver gets damaged, and even scarred, it can repair itself. So even when fatty deposits collect to the point of causing disease, the fatty deposits may fall away and the liver can become healthy again when a person loses weight.

The liver helps in the absorption of certain nutrients from foods and stores energy for later use. It also detoxifies (cleans out) anything unhealthy, such as alcohol or drugs. It produces substances that help fight infections and clot blood. The liver also loves to store fat. Excess sugar intake gets stored as fat, and when the liver tries to store too much fat, it can get sick. This is called *fatty liver disease,* and it means that fat makes up at least 10 percent of the liver.

Often, fatty liver disease isn't discovered early enough because it doesn't cause pain. Also, it can be identified only by doing a blood test, which is usually followed by an ultrasound or similar scan, and eventually a liver tissue biopsy. If fatty liver disease becomes too serious, it can lead to liver failure and may require a liver transplant to keep you alive.

Measuring the Facts

Many doctors are noticing a higher number of children with NASH. This is a new phenomenon—typically fatty liver disease doesn't appear until a person has been obese for many years, even decades.

Doctors are concerned by children whose liver looks like that of adults with cirrhosis. Until recently, that type of illness was never seen in children, but now it's becoming more common.

Research on Fatty Liver Disease

Questions remain unanswered. Why are some children, such as Hispanic males, more susceptible than the general population to liver disease? What are the predictors of the most serious forms of the disorder? Weight loss is part of the solution. For a look at recent studies, visit the American Liver Foundation at www.LiverFoundation.org.

Obstructive Sleep Apnea

Obstructive sleep apnea (OSA) is a repeated stopping of breathing during sleep. It occurs when the airway is obstructed. Common symptoms of sleep apnea are:

- loud snoring
- disrupted sleep

- gasping and choking during sleep
- daytime sleepiness and fatigue

Sleep apnea can cause high blood pressure and other cardiovascular disease, memory problems, weight gain, and headaches. In addition, untreated sleep apnea may be responsible for job impairment, poor school performance, and motor vehicle crashes.

Orthopedic Problems

The burden of excess weight on the body puts children at risk for developing orthopedic problems, such as bowing of the legs under the pressure of excess weight, knee and foot pain, scoliosis, osteoarthritis, and slipping of the thigh bone backward. These conditions can be painful and limiting for a child while making exercise more difficult.

Pseudotumor Cerebri

This rare disorder is characterized by the buildup of fluid around the brain. Common symptoms include headache, nausea, vomiting, and acute vision impairment. If left untreated, this disorder may result in permanent visual impairment such as blindness. The only remedy for this disorder is weight loss.

Depression

Obese children are more at risk for low self-esteem, withdrawal from social interaction, depression, and anxiety. A study by Jeffrey Schwimmer showed that morbidly obese adolescents view their quality of life as the same as that for children undergoing chemotherapy for cancer.

The impact of peer teasing and poor body image can be profound in adolescents. Research by Gregory Simon and colleagues suggests that being obese increases the likelihood of mood or anxiety disorders by 25 percent. Whether weight changes cause depression or depression causes weight change is up for debate.

Specific criteria exist for the diagnosis of depression, and the need for a proper assessment is critical. A psychologist is an essential part of the weight-loss team and may be the missing link to solving the food dilemmas. All of us eat for reasons besides hunger, and a mental-health professional is well suited to the essential task of behavior modification. Parental depression confers a three times greater risk of anxiety disorders and major depression in their children.

Additionally, children of depressed parents are more likely to have medical problems as well. Depression in children often manifests itself as irritability in addition to the traditional symptoms of change in sleep habits or appetite. Often mood changes can be attributed to a phase a child is going through. If you suspect depression or any mental-health concern, get a referral and get treatment.

If All Else Fails: Late-Stage Interventions

Battling obesity requires behavior modification such as evaluating your child's diet, changing eating habits, and adding daily activity. If you have tried that and still feel that little or no progress has been made in your child's struggle with obesity, keep reading.

Weight-Loss Medications

Dietary supplements are generally ineffective for true long-term weight control. Ephedra, a stimulant, was the active ingredient in popular weight-loss aids, but it was banned by the FDA due to deaths associated with the product. Since the ban, many products now contain caffeine in various forms and bitter orange, which is a cousin to ephedra.

Two medications are available to help with weight loss. They must be taken with a physician's supervision. Neither is capable of creating permanent weight loss and both have side effects.

- Xenical (orlistat) blocks fat absorption from the digestive tract and recently was approved for over-the-counter sales (Alli). Side effects can be unpleasant and include oil leakage of the unabsorbed fat from the rectum.
- Meridia (sibutramine) blocks some neurotransmitters in the brain, making people feel fuller sooner when they eat. It also increases metabolism.

Although both of these drugs have been shown to be somewhat effective, the only way to sustain long-term weight loss is to incorporate it into a healthy lifestyle: good eating habits and daily exercise.

Weight-Loss Surgery

Weight-loss surgery (its official name is bariatric surgery) is performed on the stomach, intestines, or both to help patients with morbid obesity lose weight.

However, weight-loss surgery is not a cure for obesity. Above all, patients must understand that surgery is a *tool* to help them lose weight, which can potentially reverse severe obesity-related diseases (comorbidities) in adolescents.

Rapid weight loss does occur after surgery, but at some point weight loss stops. If your child does not follow the new dietary guidelines and engage in daily exercise, he or she may not lose all the extra pounds.

What Kinds of Surgery Are There?

Weight-loss operations fall into three categories:

- *Restrictive* procedures make the stomach smaller to limit food intake.
- *Malabsorptive* techniques reduce the amount of intestine that comes in contact with food so that the body absorbs fewer calories.
- *Combination* operations utilize both restriction and malabsorption.

Gastric bypass is currently considered the "gold standard" obesity surgery. The procedure combines both restriction and malabsorption, and is the only FDA-approved procedure for adolescents.

The type of gastric bypass most frequently used is the Roux-en-Y procedure. Staples are used to permanently close off part of the stomach, leaving only a small stomach pouch, the size of an egg, for all the food eaten.

Additionally, a Y-shaped piece of tissue taken from an upper portion of the small intestine is attached to the small stomach pouch. The result is that food from the stomach pouch bypasses the initial sections of the intestine, which normally would absorb calories and nutrients from food. The amount and types of food that can be eaten after surgery are restricted. Most patients can no longer tolerate high-fat foods, high-starch foods, sweets, and carbonated beverages.

Is Surgery Right for My Child?

If your child has made real efforts to lose weight and has failed, has severe health risks, and is committed to making substantial lifestyle changes, bariatric surgery may be the next step. But just because your child is obese does not mean he or she is an appropriate candidate for surgery.

Candidates for adolescent surgery must meet strict criteria that are more conservative than those for adults. Your child will undergo a multitude of testing to identify obesity-related comorbidities. He or she also will have extensive interviews and assessments from the surgeon, behavioral therapist, dietitian, and other members of the medical team. This team collectively decides if a patient is appropriate for surgery and can stick to the rigid pre- and postoperative regimens, which include but are not limited to diet and exercise.

Criteria for Considering Adolescents for Bariatric Surgery
- has reached physical and psychological maturity
- a BMI of 40 or greater
- significant obesity-related comorbidity including, but not limited to, Type 2 diabetes, sleep apnea, hypertension, joint disease, and/or fatty liver disease
- *documented, supervised* failed attempts to lose weight

Finding a Medical Team
Bariatric surgery requires a tremendous commitment to lifestyle changes that begins long before surgery. Special support is essential for pre- and postoperative care with adolescents.

A qualified bariatric surgery program should meet the unique needs of adolescents, provide long-term follow-up care, and offer support groups for continued success after surgery. Search for a program with a multidisciplinary board consisting at a minimum of a medical director, surgical director (bariatric surgeon), pediatric anesthesiologist, psychologist, dietitian, gynecologist (if your child is a girl), and ethicist.

Life After Surgery
All surgery has potential risks. The most notable short-term risks of bariatric surgery are:

- vitamin and mineral deficiencies
- protein malnutrition, which can lead to hair loss
- nutritional deficiencies of iron, calcium, and B_{12}
- dehydration, which can lead to electrolyte imbalances
- dumping syndrome, the rapid emptying of stomach contents high in sugar or fat into the intestines, which can cause diarrhea, fainting, fatigue, headache, nausea, abdominal cramps, shakiness, difficulty concentrating, and facial flushing

Long-term consequences of bariatric surgery on adolescents are not yet known.

Nutritional complications can be avoided by following these rules:

- Eat protein first at each meal.
- Drink at least 64 ounces of liquids daily. Drink liquid before and after a meal. Limit juices and drinks high in sugar.

- No snacking between meals.
- Take a daily multivitamin and calcium supplement. Your doctor may also recommend a B-complex vitamin supplement.
- Exercise or stay active daily.

Treatment of morbid obesity in adolescents should first and foremost be based on aggressive behavioral and nutritional changes. The secret to weight loss—which really is no secret—is that calories used must be greater than calories consumed.

Weight-loss medications are occasionally effective. If all else has failed, surgery may be an option. The bottom line is that whatever program you try, healthy eating habits, behavior changes, and daily activity remain the key elements to success.

Diabetes Facts vs. Fiction

Fiction: Diabetes is caused by eating too much sugar.

Fact: In the past, before blood-glucose monitors were developed, diabetes was referred to as the sugar disease because it was diagnosed by sugar in the urine. In fact, there are two types of diabetes. Type I diabetes is the result of the immune system destroying the body's ability to produce insulin. Type 2 diabetes is the result of family history, genetics, and excess body fat. Eating too many calories, including those from sugar, increases your risk of Type 2 diabetes.

11

Successful Journeys

The ROAD to successful weight management can be challenging and hard work, but in the end can reap great rewards. The successful journeys below describe families that tried a variety of ways to conquer the weight battle. These stories represent real life. By reading these stories, we hope you will see that many of the roadblocks we all face can be overcome. Although each of these children would say it was not easy, it was well worth it.

Gwen's Story

Gwen was a skinny, energetic child, enthusiastic about gymnastics, bicycling, and the trampoline. She could eat whatever she wanted and seemed to be able to burn it right off. However, around age nine she started to fill out. Her mother didn't worry too much, as her sister went through the same pudgy phase. Her sister got taller within the year and grew right into her weight. But Gwen was different. She wasn't destined to be as tall. Her eating habits also caught up with her around this time. She was a secret eater, sneaking chips, crackers, and other snacks in her room after school. By high school she was about 30 pounds overweight. Marching band kept her weight stable during the school months, but each summer, due to inactivity and food choices, she would gain 8–10 pounds.

Gwen went from an outgoing child to a quiet, insecure teenager. She was always self-conscious about her weight and did try to diet, but it was slow and no one else in the family seemed to have to make the same sacrifices that she did. She tried counting calories and fad diets, and spent hours on the Internet looking for a pill or supplement that would take the pounds off. At eighteen, she reached her highest weight.

Luckily, Gwen had a friend with a weight problem who decided to join one of the weight-control programs with preportioned foods. With the support of her friend while living on her own in an apartment on a college campus, she found the planned program right for her. She lost 60 pounds by incorporating 60 minutes of exercise daily and a food plan that emphasized three meals and three snacks a day. Everything was portioned, and the right balance of nutrients was provided, with foods designed to keep her feeling full instead of deprived and hungry.

Her Mother's View

The hardest part was watching my daughter be miserable for so long. She wanted to lose weight, especially during high school, but she wanted a miracle cure and quick results. We went to professionals, but Gwen didn't like what she was being told. I tried to help her diet, but what worked for me didn't seem to be what she wanted or needed. The more depressed she became, the harder it was to motivate her to do anything.

I was excited when she finally found a friend and a sound program to try. Although it was expensive to join and I wasn't sure she would stick with it, I felt compelled to support her in the decision.

As I reflect back, there were so many lessons learned. Because her father and I both worked, meals were a challenge. However, our meals would have been more balanced if I had done more aggressive planning and organizing of the foods. Gwen's father came home from work first and did the cooking. He struggled with the girls each evening about what to cook, and undoubtedly keeping peace became more important than the final meal. When I planned meals, giving each girl a day to pick her favorite foods, meals were much better. However, this was not a consistent practice.

Realizing that after-school snacking was a problem, having healthier choices around the house would have been helpful. Again, this took planning, but it also meant everyone else would have to make some diet changes. As the one doing the shopping, instead of giving in to the pressure of the rest of the family members, I should have bought healthier foods and prepared them ahead of time for snacks.

Gwen tried to tell me what she needed for a successful diet: She wanted someone to fix her food and make all the decisions for her. Knowing my own struggles, I felt it was more important to learn about food so you could make better choices no matter what situation you were in. What I didn't realize was that Gwen needed the control of preportioned meals until she was successful. She couldn't deal with learning until she was happier with herself and could see that it could work. That's one of the hardest parts of parenting: asking your kids the right questions so you can understand their motivations versus wanting to provide them the answer.

Gwen's View

I really didn't like myself much all through school and wanted to be thinner. I know I have to take responsibility for my actions. I put the food in my mouth and I chose to sit and watch TV too much. My parents made rules, but not everyone had to follow them. That sometimes was my excuse for sneaking some foods. It would have been easier if there were only healthy options in the house and I didn't have to be tempted.

Even though my mom was trying to help me find the right diet, I wanted fast results and she knew I would have to diet sensibly for a while. I needed to learn that myself. I also needed to come to terms with dieting when I was ready, which didn't happen until I had tried some fads and found they don't work. I'm glad my family supported me when I was ready for the longer-term commitment.

Rewards and small goals were definitely good things. I didn't think it would be so important to celebrate the five-pound losses, but they started adding up. It was much easier to stay motivated when I felt I was going in the right direction with my weight. I'm very happy with my results thus far and know I have to make my new food and exercise choices and habits a lifelong commitment.

Marissa's Story

Marissa is sixteen years old and has struggled with her weight since her mother left her family. Her weight increased from 155 to over 215 pounds in the last year. She has a supportive dad and grandparents who are more than willing to help. Her grandparents brought her to the clinic, but her first visit to the healthcare team was less than successful. She didn't want to see the dietitian to be put on a diet. She doesn't like talking about her worries and it became clear that a therapist must become involved. During her visits with the psychologist, she opened up and discussed the real reasons her weight began to climb. She was frightened and depressed after her mother left and now realized she had been eating for comfort.

She agreed to keep a food journal and she gave her grandparents a list of foods that she wanted kept out of the house. Her grandparents helped her to grocery shop and assisted in food preparation. Although she doesn't like exercise, she agreed to walk the dog for 20 minutes per day.

Within three months, Marissa had lost 20 pounds and dropped three dress sizes. Her dad took her to buy a new outfit for school and she can now buy clothes that she likes.

Grandparents' View

We wanted Marissa to know that she was loved, so when her mother left, we bought Marissa foods that we knew she liked. She had been through a rough time and we thought cookies and ice cream would make her feel better. We learned that there were other ways to support our granddaughter. We learned that she needed some help in making good food choices, and we took her to the store. The dietitian taught us how to lower the calories in her favorite foods. We also learned that it was less about calorie counting and more about making better choices. We saw Marissa getting excited about losing weight, and we got excited too. For the holidays, she asked for a few sessions with a personal trainer, and we were happy to give this as a gift. We found a gym close to her home and she was excited about her progress.

Marissa's View

I was so sad after my mom left that I just started eating. When my grandparents took me to the doctor to lose weight, I was mad. The doctor told me about the problems associated with my weight and I got scared. I am only sixteen and could not think about having diabetes. I did not want to talk to the dietitian and I certainly didn't want a diet! But I did meet my psychologist, and she was really cool. She listened to me and we talked about how to solve problems, and after meeting with her a few times, I was ready to go back to the dietitian. She helped me to make better choices throughout the day, starting with breakfast. I stopped eating muffins and doughnuts and switched to cereal instead. My grandparents took me shopping and we got fresh fruit and vegetables. They helped me make salad and grilled some chicken for my dad and me. We ate some dinners to-gether, and most of the foods we made were really good. But losing weight is the best thing. My clothes fit better. Even though I still want to lose more weight, I feel good and the doctor told me that the early warning signs of diabetes are gone. I have learned about food, cooking, shopping—and me.

Davy's Story

Davy was a very pleasant eight-year-old who came to see Monica, a registered dietitian, in a community clinic. Davy was very concerned because some of the kids at school were making fun of him. When asked what his goals were, he responded, "to be healthy, be able to run fast on the basketball court, and not have kids laugh at me." His mother, stepfather, dad, and stepmother were also very concerned about his weight and mental well-being. His parents and stepparents, though they don't always get along, realized that they needed to come together in order to help Davy be healthier.

Davy splits his time half and half at each house. According to his parents, his eating behaviors and habits were pretty much the same in each house. He usually ate three meals plus one snack each day. Although the parents reported overall "healthy" eating habits (baked foods vs. fried; skim milk vs. whole milk), Davy was still very overweight for his age. It appeared that portion size was a big problem with both families. For example, at breakfast he had a tendency to "pile" peanut butter on waffles or a biscuit. He also ate as much meat and potatoes as his dad at dinner. His parents had already taken some steps to help with his weight, such as limiting regular soda to 1 per day, but he was drinking 2 to 3 juices a day. The parents also had a very hard time getting Davy to eat fruits or vegetables. He had no interest in them and wouldn't even try them.

Davy is very physically active, playing basketball for a very competitive league and also with his friends daily. His basketball practices are 2 days a week for 2 hours each and then 1 to 2 games each week. He has PE each day in school, but only 3 days a week do they do something that makes him sweat. Davy really liked to drink a sports drink during and after practice/games.

When they all left the office, it was understood that Davy was going to help measure out his food portions and stick to the recommended amount. He was also going to drink only diet sodas or sugar-free beverages—meaning no juice (Davy was not happy about this but did agree to it). He was going to try and drink 6 to 8 cups of water each day and was allowed a 12-ounce sports drink after one of his basketball games each week. Davy and Monica discussed how vegetables were good for his body and also helped to make him feel full because of the fiber they provide. This was the group that was designated "2nds ONLY"—if he was still hungry after eating dinner and drinking his water, he could have seconds only from the vegetable group. Davy was also going to continue being physically active, though now he would do a few different activities to help work different muscles. He said he was going to walk around the block with his mom or dad and would ride his bike sometimes.

Monica's View

A month after seeing Davy, I received a delightful phone call from him. Davy told me that his "pants were getting much bigger." Although I could not see his face, I could tell from his voice that he was grinning from ear to ear. Davy also told me that he had been helping his mom and stepmother measure out food portions, not only for him, but for his parents too! He seemed to really enjoy that. I asked Davy about the vegetables, and he said he found out that he liked broccoli—who knew? He was so excited! I asked Davy how his basketball playing was going, and he said he felt like he was starting to run a little faster and could jump a little higher.

Mother's View

We were concerned about Davy and wanted to help him be happy with himself. We realized when we talked with the dietitian just how important it was that we make changes as a family. I was so happy when Davy called the dietitian with his update and also reported that he had lost about 8 pounds in the month since we had seen her. Both sets of parents are very pleased with his progress and ALL of our new healthy lifestyle.

Davy is due for another visit with Monica in about four weeks. There is no doubt, with the changes the family has made TOGETHER, and our love and support, Davy is going to be just fine. We were able to stop the weight gain before it became a problem that was completely out of control. Davy is so excited that he has even invited Monica to come watch one of his basketball games.

All of these stories stress the importance of role-modeling, organizing the choices your family makes regarding food and exercise, making healthy foods accessible, and deciding to take the ROAD to better health. As you and your family begin this journey, the team at Texas Children's Hospital wishes you safe passage on the ROAD to success.

PART IV

• • •

Family Recipes

12

• • •

Breakfasts

Breakfast Burrito

8 egg whites or 1 cup egg
   substitute
2 whole eggs
Nonstick cooking spray
4 low-fat flour tortillas
½ cup low-fat Monterey Jack
   cheese

1 large tomato, chopped
1 medium onion, chopped
¼ green or red bell pepper, chopped
½ avocado, diced
Salsa
Sliced olives
½ cup meat (optional)

1. Beat together egg whites and eggs.
2. Spray a frying pan with nonstick cooking spray and scramble the eggs.
3. Warm the tortillas in the microwave. Fill each with one-quarter of the eggs and your choice of ingredients. Fold into a burrito.

Serving size: 1 burrito; serves 4

Calories: 252
Carbohydrate: 27 grams
Protein: 16 grams
Fat: 9 grams

Fiber: 1 gram
Sodium: 493 milligrams
Cholesterol: 169 milligrams

Nutrition Tip: Substituting egg whites for whole eggs reduces the fat and calories. In this recipe, many of the whole eggs were replaced with an egg white substitute, saving 80 calories per serving.

Generally you can substitute 2 egg whites for every whole egg. This substitution may make baked goods less tender. To compensate, add 1 teaspoon of oil per egg called for in a recipe.

Chef's Cinnamon Toast

2 tablespoons reduced-fat
    margarine
2 tablespoons powdered sugar

½ teaspoon ground cinnamon
3 slices wheat bread

1. Preheat oven to 350°F.
2. Place softened margarine in a small mixing bowl. Mix in powdered sugar and cinnamon. Use a rubber spatula to mix the ingredients until they are a smooth paste.
3. Spread the cinnamon mixture equally on the 3 slices of bread. Place in the oven until the topping is brown and bubbly, about 3 minutes.
4. Allow toast to cool for 2–3 minutes before eating.

Serving size: 1 slice; serves 3

Calories: 102
Carbohydrate: 17 grams
Protein: 2 grams
Fat: 3 grams

Fiber: 1 gram
Sodium: 178 milligrams
Cholesterol: 0 milligrams

Nutrition Tip: Eating healthier is also about incorporating all the important nutrients. Fiber not only helps decrease fat absorption but also helps you feel full longer. Whole wheat is just one of many whole grains we need to incorporate into our diets. When choosing a whole-grain product, select foods that name one of the following whole-grain ingredients *first* on the label's ingredients list:

- brown rice
- wild rice
- graham flour

- whole-grain corn
- whole oats
- whole wheat

- oatmeal
- bulgur
- rye

Foods labeled "multi-grain," "stone-ground," "100% wheat," "cracked wheat," "seven-grain," or "bran" are usually *not* whole-grain products.

Color is not an indication of a whole grain. Bread can be brown because of molasses or other added ingredients. Read the ingredients list to see if it is a whole grain.

Fruit Scones

3 cups all-purpose flour
⅓ cup sugar
1 tablespoon baking
    powder
½ teaspoon baking soda
¼ teaspoon salt
6 tablespoons butter,
    chilled and cut into 6
    pieces

⅓ cup dried apricots,
    chopped
⅓ cup dried cranberries
    (Craisins)
⅔ cup low-fat buttermilk
2 teaspoons orange rind,
    grated
1 large egg
1 egg white

1. Preheat oven to 375°F.
2. Combine dry ingredients and butter with a hand mixer or in a food processor until it resembles coarse cornmeal.
3. Stir in apricots and cranberries.
4. Combine buttermilk, orange rind, egg, and egg white, then add to flour mixture, stirring just until moist.
5. Turn dough out onto a lightly floured surface and knead lightly with floured hands about four times. Roll out dough to 1¼" thickness. Cut circles with 2" cookie cutter or a glass.
6. Place scones on baking sheet, sprinkle with sugar, and bake 10–12 minutes or until lightly brown.

Serving size: 1 scone; makes 25 scones

Calories: 106
Carbohydrate: 17 grams
Protein: 2 grams
Fat: 4 grams

Fiber: 1 gram
Sodium: 121 milligrams
Cholesterol: 17 milligrams

Nutrition Tip: Most breakfast pastries are high in fat and calories. The benefit of a treat like this is that there is no need for added butter as a topping. It is higher in complex carbohydrates than doughnuts and the fruit adds fiber and vitamins.

These scones can be frozen. Just reheat in the microwave or a conventional oven.

13

• • •

Soups and Main Dishes

Easy Alphabet Soup

1 stalk celery chopped
½ medium onion, chopped
2 cups frozen mixed
    vegetables (or fresh
    vegetables such as
    chopped carrots, peas,
    green beans, etc.)
¼ teaspoon dried thyme
6 cups fat-free chicken broth

1 bay leaf
1 cup uncooked alphabet
    macaroni
2 (5-ounce) cans chunk
    chicken (or use 2–3
    cooked boneless chicken
    breasts, cut in small
    pieces)
Salt and pepper (optional)

1. Cook macaroni according to package directions for al dente. Don't over-cook.
2. Meanwhile, in a large pot, place celery, onion, mixed vegetables, thyme, chicken broth, and bay leaf. Bring mixture to a boil over medium heat. Simmer 12–15 minutes, until vegetables are tender.
3. Combine macaroni and vegetables. Add chicken. Cook about 2 minutes until chicken is heated. Remove bay leaf. Add salt and pepper to taste.

Serving size: 1½ cups; serves 8

Calories: 134
Carbohydrate: 17 grams
Protein: 12 grams
Fat: 2 grams

Fiber: 3 grams
Sodium: 85 milligrams
Cholesterol: 21 milligrams

Nutrition Tip: Many people prefer fresh foods to processed. Processed foods usually contain a lot of sodium. The new dietary guidelines recommend a much lower sodium intake than previously encouraged. Blending some scratch cooking with convenience foods is a good way to reduce your family's intake of salt as well as teach your children different food flavors. Most recipes like this say to salt and pepper "to taste." Season your foods with other herbs and spices, then taste the food before adding salt. Just because one family member likes salty foods doesn't mean everyone does, or needs to get that habit started.

Broccoli-Cheese Soup

1½ pounds fresh or frozen
    broccoli, cut up
2 cups low-fat or skim milk
2 cups water
1 pound low-fat pasteurized
    processed cheese loaf, cut
    into 1-inch cubes

¾ teaspoon salt
½ cup cornstarch
1 cup cold water
Ground black pepper
    (optional)

1. Steam broccoli until tender, or microwave on high power about 6 minutes.
2. Combine milk, 2 cups water, cheese, and salt in a microwave-safe bowl. Microwave until cheese is melted, about 6 minutes, stirring at 1-minute intervals, or melt in a saucepan on the stove over medium heat for about 5 minutes. Do not let it boil, or cheese will curdle.
3. Place broccoli and cheese mixture in a large saucepan.
4. Mix cornstarch and cold water in small bowl. Stir into cheese mixture and cook over medium heat, stirring constantly, until thickened and heated through.
5. Top with ground pepper, if desired.

Serving size: 1 cup; serves 6–8

Calories: 216
Carbohydrate: 19 grams
Protein: 17 grams
Fat: 8 grams

Fiber: 3 grams
Sodium: 573 milligrams
Cholesterol: 21 milligrams

Nutrition Tip: Soups can be a great start to any meal or the entire meal itself. To make it fun, try a variety of garnishes to add color and eye appeal. Some healthy ideas include shredded carrots, minced fresh herbs, grated low-fat cheese, low-fat croutons, snow peas, or a dollop of low-fat yogurt.

Not all soups are the same. Broth-based soups tend to be lower in calories than milk- or cream-based soups. Making your own and using lower-fat ingredients like this recipe can significantly reduce calories. Soup is also a good way to fill up before a meal. By adding the soup appetizer, you may be less likely to want seconds of higher-calorie foods.

Terry's Gumbo

⅓ cup corn oil
½–⅔ cup all-purpose flour
1 cup chopped onion
1 cup chopped celery
1 cup chopped green bell
    pepper
1 teaspoon garlic powder
2 teaspoons dried parsley
1 quart fat-free, reduced-
    sodium beef or chicken
    broth
1½ cups canned chopped
    tomatoes, low-sodium

1 cup tomato sauce
1 teaspoon creole
    seasoning
Minced fresh garlic clove
2 teaspoons low-sodium
    chicken bouillon
2 cups water
Salt to taste
1 cup chopped okra
1 pound cooked or raw shrimp,
    chicken, or sausage (or
    combination) (if desired)

1. Mix corn oil and flour in a heavy pot and cook over medium heat until light brown (caramel color).
2. Mix onion, celery, pepper, garlic, and parsley into the roux (flour and oil mixture) and cook until soft, not brown.
3. Add broth, tomatoes, tomato sauce, creole seasoning, garlic powder, chicken bouillon, salt (if desired), and water. Stir until roux is smooth and cook over low-medium heat for 2 hours.
4. Add okra and cooked meat (if desired). Cook until okra is done, about 5 minutes. Extend cooking time if using raw meat or shrimp.

Nutrition Tip: Roux gives gumbo its distinctive flavor. Commercial roux is available in a jar. Another time-saving trick, so you can make your own soups and gumbos, is purchasing chopped frozen vegetables. To keep the fat content down, use chicken or shrimp instead of sausage.

Serving size: 1 cup; serves 12

Calories: 151

Carbohydrate: 10 grams

Protein: 14 grams

Fat: 6 grams

Fiber: 2 grams

Sodium: 348 milligrams

Cholesterol: 32 milligrams

Apple Crunch Salad

1 (3-ounce) package sugar-free strawberry (or other fruit) gelatin

1 cup boiling water

⅛ teaspoon cinnamon

¾ cup cold water

½ cup peeled and chopped apple

1 cup water

1 teaspoon lemon juice

¼ cup celery

2 tablespoons chopped nuts

1. Dissolve gelatin in boiling water, stirring well.
2. Mix cinnamon with cold water.
3. Combine cinnamon mixture and gelatin. Stir.
4. Chill until thickened, about 1 hour.
5. Soak apples in water and lemon juice.
6. Drain apples and fold into gelatin mixture. Fold in celery and nuts.
7. Divide the gelatin into 5 small bowls or goblet-type wineglasses. Chill until firm, about 4 hours.

Serving size: ½ cup; serves 5

Calories: 32 (14 without nuts)

Carbohydrate: 3 grams

Fat: 2 grams

Fiber: 1 gram

Sodium: 56 milligrams

Cholesterol: 0 milligrams

Nutrition Tip: This is a great recipe to add fruits and introduce textures to your children. Apples, pears (check out the variety of apples and pears in your grocery store), or other crunchy fruits work well.

Sugar-free Jell-O is a very low-calorie way to enjoy a sweet without guilt. Look at the difference for ½ cup of regular Jell-O versus sugar-free Jell-O:

regular Jell-O: 130 calories   sugar-free Jell-O: 10 calories

Substitute sugar free for any of your traditional Jell-O recipes.

Macaroni and Cheese

2 cups dry elbow macaroni,
   or pasta shape your
   children choose
2 tablespoons nonfat, dry
   milk
2 tablespoons flour

1 tablespoon margarine
1¼ cups boiling water
3 cups grated reduced-fat
   American cheese, divided
¼ teaspoon salt
Nonstick cooking spray

1. Preheat oven to 350°F.
2. Cook macaroni according to package directions.
3. Meanwhile, mix dry milk, flour, and margarine in a large mixing bowl. Gradually add boiling water, beating constantly. Add 1½ cups cheese and continue beating until smooth and creamy.
4. Stir in macaroni, 1 cup cheese, and salt. Transfer to a 2-quart baking dish sprayed with nonstick cooking spray. Cover with foil and bake 25 minutes.
5. Remove foil and sprinkle with remaining ½ cup cheese. Bake 1 minute longer or until cheese melts.

Serving size: 1 cup; serves 8

Calories: 182
Carbohydrate: 24 grams
Protein: 17 grams
Fat: 2 grams

Fiber: 1 gram
Sodium: 395 milligrams
Cholesterol: 0 milligrams

Broccoli-Cheese Casserole

1 cup water
1 cup instant rice
1 tablespoon olive oil
¼ cup chopped onion
¼ cup chopped celery
1 (10¾-ounce) can reduced-
   fat cream of mushroom
   soup

1 (10¾-ounce) can reduced-
   fat cream of celery soup
1 (10-ounce) package frozen
   chopped broccoli, thawed
½ cup diced, reduced-fat,
   processed American
   cheese
Nonstick cooking spray

1. Preheat oven to 350°F.
2. Bring water and salt to a boil in a saucepan. Add rice. Cover and remove from heat. Let it sit for 5 minutes.
3. Heat olive oil in a small skillet. Sauté onion and celery until tender.
4. Combine rice, celery, soups, broccoli, and cheese in a large mixing bowl. Pour into a 1½-quart casserole dish, sprayed with nonstick cooking spray. Bake for 1 hour.

Serving size: 1 cup; serves 6

Calories: 195
Carbohydrate: 25 grams
Protein: 8 grams
Fat: 7 grams

Fiber: 3 grams
Sodium: 853 milligrams
Cholesterol: 11 milligrams

(continued)

(*continued*)
When people diet, they can quickly start cutting out the foods that are rich in needed nutrients. That's why the best approach is to find tasty, healthy recipes rich in vitamins and minerals. Calcium-rich foods and weight-bearing exercise at least three times a week make for stronger bones. Another good reason to exercise!

Cheese Enchiladas

10 (6-inch) corn tortillas
2 (10-ounce) cans mild
enchilada sauce

2 cups shredded reduced-fat Colby,
Jack, cheddar, or American cheese
Nonstick cooking spray

1. Preheat oven to 350°F.
2. Wrap tortillas in plastic wrap. Microwave 1 minute to soften.
3. Dip each tortilla in enchilada sauce.
4. Spoon about 2 tablespoons of cheese down center of each tortilla. Roll up and place seam side down in a 13"×9" baking dish sprayed with nonstick cooking spray.
5. Pour remaining enchilada sauce over filled enchiladas. Sprinkle with remaining cheese. Bake for 20–25 minutes.

Serving size: 2 enchiladas; serves 5

Calories: 234
Carbohydrate: 31 grams
Protein: 19 grams
Fat: 4 grams

Fiber: 3 grams
Sodium: 409 milligrams
Cholesterol: 0 milligrams

Nutrition Tip: Ever go to a restaurant and order enchiladas, only to get three large ones? It's important early on to learn what a proper portion size is. In this recipe, a serving is two. Watch what you serve with enchiladas. Instead of rice, chips, or *queso,* serve fat-free refried beans, jicama strips, *pico de gallo,* or nopalitos.

Easy Cheese Lasagna

9 uncooked lasagna noodles
1 (15-ounce) can tomato
   sauce
1 (14-ounce) jar low-fat
   spaghetti sauce
16 ounces cottage cheese, 1%
   or nonfat

½ cup grated, part skim Parmesan
   cheese
8 ounces low-fat or fat-free
   mozzarella cheese,
   shredded
Nonstick cooking spray

1. Preheat oven to 350°F.
2. In a small bowl, combine tomato and spaghetti sauces.
3. In another bowl, combine the cottage and Parmesan cheeses.
4. Spray a 13"×9" baking pan with nonstick spray. Place 3 uncooked noodles on the bottom of the pan. Cover with ⅓ of the sauce, ⅓ of the cottage cheese–parmesan mixture, and ⅓ of the mozzarella. Repeat this layering two more times with noodles, sauce, and cheese. Cover dish tightly with foil.
5. Bake for 1 hour. Let stand 15 minutes before serving.

Serving size: 4"×3" square; serves 8

Calories: 186
Carbohydrate: 14 grams
Protein: 24 grams
Fat: 3 grams

Fiber: 2 grams
Sodium: 1000 milligrams
Cholesterol: 42 milligrams

Nutrition Tip: Cottage cheese comes in a variety of fat content levels from low or nonfat (0–1%) to higher fat (4%). The cheese is what makes the texture of this dish; higher-fat cheeses only add calories and are not necessary. This recipe uses the lower-fat cheeses Parmesan and mozzarella, which are made from part-skim milk.

Chinese Noodle Casserole

1 pound extra-lean ground
    meat
1 medium onion, cut in thin
    slices and separated into
    rings
Nonstick cooking spray
1 (10½-ounce) can reduced-
    fat cream of mushroom
    soup

1 (10½-ounce) can reduced-
    fat cream of chicken
    soup
1 can sliced water chestnuts,
    drained
1 large can Chinese noodles,
    divided
1 can Chinese vegetables,
    drained

1. Preheat oven to 350°F.
2. Sauté ground meat and onion in a nonstick pan until meat is cooked and onion is transparent. Drain grease from meat in a colander and rinse with warm water poured from a cup.
3. Spray a 3-quart casserole dish with nonstick cooking spray. Add meat mixture, soups, water chestnuts, ½ can Chinese noodles, and Chinese vegetables. Mix to combine. Top with remaining Chinese noodles. Wipe inside rim of the casserole dish with paper towel.
4. Cover and bake for 45 minutes.

Serving size: ⅛ of casserole; serves 8

Calories: 250
Carbohydrate: 17 grams
Protein: 14 grams
Fat: 14 grams

Fiber: 2 grams
Sodium: 664 milligrams
Cholesterol: 41 milligrams

Nutrition Tip: Check the numbers when buying ground meat. The higher the percent, the lower the fat content. Extralean ground beef (95%) has about 25% less fat than regular ground beef (70%). You may also see other names for ground beef. Ground round is the leanest, followed by ground sirloin, ground chuck, and then regular ground beef. If you do use regular ground beef, be sure to drain it well and rinse it with hot water after it is cooked to remove as much fat as possible.

Sloppy Joes

1 pound ground beef, lean	1 teaspoon cider vinegar
1 medium onion, diced	1 teaspoon sugar
¼ cup ketchup	½ cup barbecue sauce
2 tablespoons chili sauce	6 whole wheat hamburger
1 teaspoon yellow mustard	buns

1. Brown meat and onions in a large skillet over medium-high heat. Pour off fat.
2. Add all other ingredients, except buns, mixing well. Reduce heat and simmer 20–30 minutes, uncovered.
3. Spoon onto hamburger buns and serve immediately.

Serving size: 1 sandwich; serves 6

Calories: 274	Fiber: 4 grams
Carbohydrate: 39 grams	Sodium: 915 milligrams
Protein: 23 grams	Cholesterol: 30 milligrams
Fat: 3 grams	

Nutrition Tip: Ever wonder how to use the nutritional information found on recipes? You will notice the recipes have the nutrient values indicated for calories, fat, protein, cholesterol, sodium, carbohydrate, and fiber. To understand how much of these nutrients you should normally eat, you can use the standard amounts listed on the *Nutrition Facts* label on any packaged food item. The Food and Drug Administration has set standards for 2000 and 2500 calorie diets for the nutrients.

You may need less or more of the indicated amounts depending on your age, weight, and activity level. Most children and some adults will need less than 2000 per day, while an active, growing teenager may need quite a bit more.

The standard nutrient amounts listed on the *Nutrition Facts* label for a 2000 calorie per day diet are:

Calories- 2000
Total Fat- Less than 65 grams
Cholesterol- Less than 300 milligrams
Sodium- Less than 2400 milligrams
Total Carbohydrate- 300 grams
Dietary Fiber- 25 grams

Beef Tortilla Pizza

1 pound extra-lean ground
    beef
1 medium onion,
    chopped
1 teaspoon Italian
    seasoning
1 teaspoon salt

6 (6-inch) flour tortillas
Olive oil
1 medium tomato, chopped
1 cup part-skim mozzarella
    cheese, shredded
¼ cup dried basil (optional)

1. Preheat oven to 400°F.
2. Brown ground beef and onion in skillet over medium heat until done. Drain meat mixture in colander, rinsing with hot water poured from a cup. Wipe grease from skillet. Return mixture to pan.
3. Stir in Italian seasoning and salt.
4. Lightly brush tortillas with olive oil. Place on a large baking sheet and bake for 3 minutes.
5. Spoon beef mixture evenly over top of each tortilla. Top with equal amounts of tomato. Sprinkle with cheese. Sprinkle basil on top, if desired.
6. Return to oven and bake 6–8 minutes, or until tortillas are lightly browned.

Serving size: 1 pizza; serves 6

Calories: 334
Carbohydrate: 24 grams
Protein: 24 grams
Fat: 16 grams

Fiber: 2 grams
Sodium: 746 milligrams
Cholesterol: 60 milligrams

Nutrition Tip: Flour tortillas can be high in fat and low in fiber. Look for fat-free or whole wheat tortillas to reduce fat and add a source of fiber. Flavored tortillas can also add variety and flavor.

Oven-Fried Chicken Tenders

½ cup flour
½ cup low-fat milk
2 tablespoons honey
3 cups corn or wheat flaked
   cereal

1 pound boneless, skinless
   chicken breasts
½ teaspoon seasoned salt
Nonstick cooking spray

1. Preheat oven to 350°F.
2. Place flour in small bowl. Place milk and honey in another small bowl and blend well. Crush cereal and place in a third small bowl.
3. Rinse and dry chicken breasts. Cut each breast into 3 strips or tenders. Season with seasoned salt.
4. Dip each strip in flour to coat. Then dip the strip into milk-honey mixture, coating well. Then roll strip in cereal, coating well.
5. Place each strip on a cookie sheet sprayed with nonstick cooking spray.
6. Bake about 20–30 minutes, or until juices run clear when pierced.

Serving size: 2 tenders; serves 6

Calories: 214
Carbohydrate: 20 grams
Protein: 20 grams
Fat: 6 grams

Fiber: 1 gram
Sodium: 216 milligrams
Cholesterol: 47 milligrams

Nutrition Tip: Did you know that the light meat (breast) of chicken or turkey has about 30 percent less fat than the dark meat? Removing the skin from chicken also significantly reduces the fat content.

As you look at your recipes, consider using ground turkey breast instead of ground beef. Ground turkey breast works great in burgers and casseroles, and is about 99 percent fat free.

Angel Hair Pasta with Chicken

1 (12-ounce) box angel hair
   pasta (3 cups cooked)
2 tablespoons olive oil
2 boneless, skinless chicken
   breast halves (cut into 1"-
   thick cubes)
1–2 carrots, sliced diagonally
   (¼" pieces)

1 (10-ounce) bag frozen
   broccoli florets, thawed
1 clove garlic, minced
⅔ cup low-sodium chicken
   broth
1 teaspoon dried basil
¼ cup grated Parmesan
   cheese

1. Cook pasta according to package directions. (Angel hair pasta cooks quickly. Don't overcook.)
2. Heat 1 tablespoon olive oil in a skillet over medium heat. Add chicken. Cook, stirring, until chicken is cooked through, about 5 minutes. Remove from skillet and drain on paper towels.
3. Heat the remaining oil in same skillet. Add carrots and cook, stirring, for 4 minutes.
4. Add broccoli and garlic to skillet. Cook, stirring, for 2 minutes longer.
5. Add chicken broth, basil, and Parmesan to skillet. Stir to combine.
6. Return chicken to skillet. Reduce heat and simmer for 4 minutes.
7. Spoon chicken mixture over cooked pasta.

Serving size: 1½ cups; serves 6

Calories: 233
Carbohydrate: 19 grams
Protein: 26 grams
Fat: 5 grams

Fiber: 2 grams
Sodium: 196 milligrams
Cholesterol: 73 milligrams

Nutrition Tip: To make cooking from scratch much easier, seasonings like garlic or onions can be chopped and stored in the refrigerator or freezer. You can also cook large batches of pasta ahead of time and freeze them in smaller batches for one recipe. Sturdier pastas like spaghetti and macaroni freeze best. Just pull out enough for your dinner and reheat. You can reheat small batches of pasta in the microwave oven, in a colander by pouring boiling water over it, or cook it again for 1–2 minutes in a pot of boiling water and drain. Cooking ahead and reheating the pasta saves you 15 minutes of preparation time.

Nutrition Tip: Lower-fat cheese has fewer calories than its whole-milk counterpart. To know you are getting a low-fat cheese, read the label and look for dry-curd or low-fat cottage cheese, low-fat natural cheese, or processed cheese made with nonfat or low-fat milk with no more than 3 grams of fat and no more than 2 grams of saturated fat per ounce.

Chicken or Turkey Tetrazzini

1 pound boneless, skinless
   chicken or turkey breast,
   diced in 1" cubes
½ cup chopped onion
¾ shredded reduced-fat sharp
   cheddar cheese
1 can reduced-fat cream of
   mushroom soup

2 cups spaghetti, cooked
   (5 ounces, uncooked)
2 tablespoons dried
   parsley
1 jar pimientos, diced
⅛ teaspoon black pepper
1¾ cup water

1. Heat a large nonstick skillet or saucepan over medium-high heat. Add diced chicken or turkey and onion. Sauté 3 minutes, or until meat is cooked and onion is tender.
2. Stir in water, cheese, and soup. Reduce heat to low and cook 4 minutes, or until cheese melts, stirring until mixture is smooth.
3. Stir in pasta, parsley, pimientos, and pepper. Cook until thoroughly heated.

Serving size: 1 cup; serves 6

Calories: 197
Carbohydrate: 17 grams
Protein: 19 grams
Fat: 5 grams

Fiber: 1 gram
Sodium: 363 milligrams
Cholesterol: 47 milligrams

Crisp Oven-Fried Chicken

1½ cups mashed potato flakes
1 teaspoon seasoned salt
¾ teaspoon paprika
½ teaspoon chopped
   garlic
¼ teaspoon pepper

¼ teaspoon reduced-fat
   margarine
1 tablespoon water
2 egg whites
8 pieces boneless, skinless
   chicken breasts (3 pounds)

Nutrition Tip: Breading can take on many different flavors if you are creative with the dipping combinations. Crushed cereals, crackers, baked chips can all be used for chicken. Since the egg mixture helps the coating adhere, reducing the calories by using only the egg whites and lower-fat margarines does not affect the flavor. You can make chicken nuggets with this recipe also. A baked nugget has fewer calories than its fast-food counterpart.

To avoid resorting to fast-food restaurants, have your own fast food around. Prepare individual servings of nuggets by breading and then freezing one portion per individual freezer bag. Bake at 400°F without thawing.

Make your own nugget shapes. Flatten chicken breasts using a rolling pin. Cut into squares, diamonds, or other fun shapes. Use the leftover scraps in a chicken casserole or salad.

1. Preheat oven to 400°F.
2. In a large bowl, combine potato flakes, seasoned salt, paprika, garlic, and pepper. Add margarine. Mix well.
3. In medium bowl, beat water with egg whites. Dip chicken pieces in egg mixture. Then coat all sides with potato flake mixture.
4. Place chicken in ungreased 13"×9" pan. Bake uncovered for 25–30 minutes, or until chicken is fork tender and juices run clear.

Serving size: 1 chicken breast; serves 8

Calories: 214
Carbohydrate: 8 grams
Protein: 28 grams
Fat: 7 grams

Fiber: 7 grams
Sodium: 165 milligrams
Cholesterol: 66 milligrams

Tuna Canoes

¼ cup nonfat plain
    yogurt
2 tablespoons fat-free
    mayonnaise
1 teaspoon mustard
¼ teaspoon dried dill
    weed

1 (6-ounce) can water-packed
    tuna, drained
⅓ cup chopped or shredded
    carrot
2 hot dog buns split
½ cup shredded low-fat
    cheddar cheese

Nutrition Tip: Vegetables can be added to foods in a variety of ways. In this recipe, the shredded carrots not only give color and texture but also added nutrients. Try vegetables such as zucchini or yellow squash cut in julienne strips. You can also use chicken instead of tuna. Use other fun food such as Craisins for color or wheat germ for crunch.

Try whole wheat buns, or put this tuna spread in a pita pocket or other low-fat bread. You can even add various greens, including cabbage or leaf lettuce.

1. Mix together yogurt, mayonnaise, mustard, and dill weed in a medium mixing bowl.
2. Stir in tuna and carrot. Mix well.
3. Hollow out hot dog buns with a fork.
4. Sprinkle cheese into hollowed-out buns. Spoon tuna mixture over cheese.

Serving size: 1 canoe (½ bun); serves 4

Calories: 166
Carbohydrate: 18 grams
Protein: 19 grams
Fat: 2 grams

Fiber: 1 gram
Sodium: 380 milligrams
Cholesterol: 27 milligrams

Sesame-Seared Salmon

2 tablespoons sesame seeds
1¼ teaspoons olive oil
4 salmon fillets, 1" thick, 4 ounces each

1¼ tablespoons honey
2½ teaspoons soy sauce
¼ teaspoon ground ginger

1. Place sesame seeds in a nonstick skillet and sauté until golden, about 30 seconds. Remove to a plate and set aside.
2. Heat olive oil in the same skillet on medium-high. Add salmon and sauté 5 minutes.
3. Turn salmon; sauté 3–5 more minutes, or until fish flakes easily when tested with a fork.
4. Mix together honey, soy sauce, and ginger in a small bowl.
5. Remove skillet from heat. Spoon sauce over salmon and warm in skillet 30 seconds.
6. Sprinkle with sesame seeds.

Calories: 205

Carbohydrate: 6 grams

Protein: 25 grams

Fat: 9 grams

Fiber: 0 grams

Sodium: 47 milligrams

Cholesterol: 51 milligrams

Nutrition Tip: Salmon is a rich source of omega-3 fatty acids. The American Heart Association recommends eating fish (particularly fatty fish) at least two times a week. Salmon is a higher-fat fish, but it doesn't have the high saturated fats of high-fat meats. Omega-3 fatty acids have many good health benefits and may help reduce the risk of heart disease.

Cheesy Catfish

2 egg whites

1 tablespoon skim milk

¾ cup grated Parmesan
   cheese

1¼ cups all-purpose flour

1½ cups ground black pepper

1 teaspoon paprika

8 catfish fillets, 4
   ounces each

1. Preheat oven to 350°F.
2. Beat the eggs together with the milk in a medium bowl. In another bowl, stir together the cheese, flour, pepper, and paprika.
3. Dip catfish in the egg and milk mixture, then in the cheese mixture until coated.
4. Arrange fish in a single layer in a 9" × 13" baking dish. Bake 15 minutes, or until golden brown.

Serving size: 1 fillet; serves 8

Calories: 220

Carbohydrate: 16 grams

Protein: 25 grams

Fat: 6 grams

Fiber: 1 gram

Sodium: 204 milligrams

Cholesterol: 72 milligrams

Nutrition Tip: Fish is a lower-fat protein source than many other animal products. Thus lightly battered fish baked in an oven can produce a quality low-fat entrée and save many calories.

Just look at the difference between this baked catfish and the more traditional fried version: 220 calories a serving compared to fried catfish at 260 calories per 4-ounce serving.

The coating on this fish uses low-fat items like egg whites, skim milk, and Parmesan cheese, together with the spice of pepper and paprika. Other lower-fat, mild-flavored fish to try with children are tilapia, orange roughy, and flounder.

Cheesy Tuna-Noodle Casserole

1 (12-ounce) box large pasta
   shells
2 tablespoons olive oil
¼ cup chopped onion
¼ cup chopped green bell
   pepper
¼ cup chopped red bell
   pepper

1 (11-ounce) can low-fat
   cream of cheddar soup
1 (6-ounce) can tuna, packed
   in water, drained
¼ cup skim or 1% milk
Ground pepper to taste
¼ cup Italian-seasoned bread
   crumbs
Nonstick cooking spray

1. Preheat oven to 350°F.
2. Cook pasta according to package directions.
3. While pasta is cooking, sauté olive oil, onion, and green and red peppers until tender.
4. Pour soup, tuna, milk, and pepper into the saucepan. Mix well over medium-low heat.
5. Fold the cooked pasta into the tuna mixture.
6. Pour entire mixture into a 2-quart casserole sprayed with nonstick cooking spray. Sprinkle bread crumbs over the mixture. Bake 20–30 minutes, or until the top is crisp and golden brown.

Serving size: 1¼ cups; serves 6

Calories: 344
Carbohydrate: 50 grams
Protein: 17 grams
Fat: 8 grams

Fiber: 2 grams
Sodium: 440 milligrams
Cholesterol: 15 milligrams

Nutrition Tip: Casseroles are a fun way to introduce different foods to children. You can be creative with a variety of noodle shapes to help make the dish have kid appeal, while introducing new foods.

Use water-packed tuna instead of tuna packed in oil. A 3-ounce serving of tuna in water has 85 calories; in oil, 170 calories.

Lower-fat soups also save calories over regular soups. In dishes like casseroles, the soup provides the creamy texture. The fat content is not an essential part of the recipe.

14

• • •

Side Dishes

Baked French Fries

3 medium baking
  potatoes

3 teaspoons cooking oil
Salt, if desired

1. Preheat oven to 350°F.
2. Peel potatoes and slice into large "fries."
3. Toss sliced potatoes with oil.
4. Place potatoes on a cookie sheet. Bake for about 30 minutes, or until tender.
   Stir occasionally to prevent sticking.
5. Sprinkle with salt or other seasonings, if desired.

Serves 4

Calories: 96
Carbohydrate: 19 grams
Protein: 2 grams
Fat: 3 grams

Fiber: 2 grams
Sodium: 6 milligrams
Cholesterol: 0 milligrams

Nutrition Tip: French fries are usually just that—fried. You can get rid of the extra fat calories by baking instead. A typical serving of small fast-food-restaurant-size french fries is about 210 calories. You save more than 100 calories by baking.

Leave the potato skins on to increase fiber. You also can use small red potatoes instead of baking potatoes. You can change the flavor of the potatoes by experimenting with various spices, like rosemary or garlic.

Honey-Glazed Carrots

6 medium carrots
1½ teaspoons reduced-fat margarine
1½ teaspoons honey

1. Peel carrots and cut into "coins." Place in a microwave-safe dish with 2 tablespoons water. Microwave for 5–7 minutes, or until crisp tender. Drain.
2. Melt margarine and mix with honey in a small bowl.
3. Coat carrots with honey mixture.

Serving size: ½ cup; serves 6

Calories: 70
Carbohydrate: 12 grams
Protein: 1 gram
Fat: 2 grams

Fiber: 2 grams
Sodium: 59 milligrams
Cholesterol: 0 milligrams

Grilled Vegetable Kebabs

½ cup fat-free Italian dressing
1 teaspoon dried parsley
   flakes
1 teaspoon dried basil
2 medium yellow squash, cut
   into 1" slices

2 medium onions, quartered
2 Roma tomatoes, quartered
8 medium fresh mushrooms
Nonstick cooking spray

Nutrition Tip: It's important to introduce vegetables early to your children. They probably ate their carrots when you where feeding infant foods, but now they eat what you make for yourself and the rest of the family. As the role model, you need to offer vegetables, and the entire family needs to eat them. Make the vegetables tasty and enjoyable. Carrots, like some other vegetables, are great finger foods for toddlers as you start introducing table foods. Make sure they are cooked well and are soft when introducing them to toddlers so they don't choke. You can increase firmness as the child grows.

1. Combine dressing, parsley, and basil in a small bowl.
2. Alternate squash, onions, tomatoes, and mushrooms on 4 skewers.
3. Place kebabs on a cookie sheet. Coat each kebab with dressing mixture. Cover and refrigerate for about 1 hour.
4. Coat grill rack with cooking spray. Place grill over medium coals. Place kebabs on rack and cook about 15 minutes, or until vegetables are tender. Turn frequently. Baste with additional dressing, if desired. To cook indoors, place broiler rack on lowest position and broil for 15 minutes, turning frequently.

Serving size: 1 kebab; serves 4

Calories: 48

Carbohydrate: 10 grams

Protein: 2 grams

Fat: 0 grams

Fiber: 2 grams

Sodium: 303 milligrams

Cholesterol: 0 milligrams

Bean Dip

1 (16-ounce) can black beans or pinto beans, rinsed and drained

¾ cup mild salsa

¼ cup fat-free sour cream

Chopped tomato (optional)

1. Blend beans, salsa, and sour cream in a blender or food processor until smooth.
2. Top with chopped tomato, if desired.

Nutrition Tip: Ever wonder about the difference among fat free, low fat, and reduced fat?

- Fat free means little or no fat is in the product. If there is any fat, the amount is so small it probably won't have an effect on your body.
- Low fat means the product has 3 grams or less of fat per serving.
- Reduced fat means the product has at least 25 percent less fat than regular.

Although it's important to lower fat, remember that many low-fat items are higher in carbohydrates and sugars. Check the calories too.

Serving size: ¼ cup; makes 6 servings

Calories: 64

Fiber: 3 grams

Carbohydrate: 11 grams

Sodium: 421 milligrams

Protein: 5 grams

Cholesterol: 0 milligrams

Fat: 0 grams

Nutrition Tip: Beans are a rich source of fiber, as well as many nutrients and inexpensive protein.

Cooking dry beans is very easy with just a little preplanning. Bring water to a boil and the let the beans soak in hot water for 1–4 hours, depending on the variety. To reduce gas, rinse the beans and finish cooking them in fresh water. It takes about 6 cups of water for each pound of beans you cook.

SERVING SUGGESTIONS:

The dip may be used for nachos, tostadas, or burritos.

Nachos: Bake a corn tortilla at 350°F until crisp. Top with bean dip and grated cheese. Broil until cheese is melted.

Burritos: Cover an 8"-flour tortilla with plastic wrap and microwave 20–30 seconds until soft. Top with ¼ cup bean dip, grated cheese, chopped tomatoes, and fat-free sour cream.

Vegetable Squares

1 (8-ounce) can refrigerated
  crescent rolls

4 ounces fat-free cream
  cheese, softened

¼ cup fat-free sour cream

1 teaspoon dill weed

½ teaspoon garlic powder

Broccoli and cauliflower
  florets

Cucumber and zucchini
  slices

Carrot and radishes, thinly
  sliced

Parsley flakes

1. Preheat oven to 375°F. Separate dough into 4 long rectangles. Place rectangles crosswise on a large cookie sheet. Firmly press perforations to seal. Bake for about 15 minutes, until golden brown. Cool completely.
2. Combine cream cheese, sour cream, dill weed and garlic powder in a small bowl. Blend until smooth. Spread evenly over cooled crust. Cover and refrigerate for 2 hours.
3. Cut into 30 squares. Top with a variety of vegetables and sprinkle with parsley flakes.

Serving size: 3 squares; serves 10

Calories: 105	Fiber: 0.4 gram
Carbohydrate: 1 gram	Sodium: 241 milligrams
Protein: 4 grams	Cholesterol: 1 milligram
Fat: 5 grams	

Chili con Queso

1 pound fat-free pasteurized, processed cheese product cut in 1-inch cubes

1 (14½-ounce) can chopped tomatoes, with green chilis

½ medium onion, chopped (optional)

1 teaspoon chili powder (optional)

¼ teaspoon ground cumin (optional)

Nutrition Tip: Cheese is made from milk and is a great source of calcium. But it can also be high in fat, particularly saturated fat. To get the benefits of all the nutrients and for the added flavor, look for lower-fat cheeses. Varieties include low-fat ricotta, part-skim mozzarella, or, as in the case of this recipe, many of the reduced-fat processed cheeses. As a rule of thumb, any cheese made with skim milk has less fat and the fat-reduced blends are 50–75 percent less fat than their whole-milk counterparts.

Here's another tip: Serve this with vegetables instead of chips. Using cheese to flavor vegetables is one way to get your children to eat them more often. It also teaches them to avoid higher-calorie snack foods.

1. Combine all ingredients in a 1-quart microwave-proof bowl.
2. Cover with wax paper or vented plastic wrap.
3. Microwave on high 4 minutes, or until cheese melts, stirring every 60 seconds, or combine all ingredients in a 2-quart saucepan. Heat over low heat until cheese melts, stirring constantly.
4. Serve with baked or low-fat chips or fresh vegetables. Count chips as a serving from the grain/starch food group.

Serving size: ¼ cup; serves 10

Calories: 79
Carbohydrate: 7 grams
Protein: 13 grams
Fat: 0.1 gram

Fiber: 0.25 gram
Sodium: 757 milligrams
Cholesterol: 0 milligrams

Pizza Snacks

8 rice cakes
½ cup pizza or spaghetti
    sauce
8 ounces low-fat mozzarella
    cheese, grated

2 tablespoons Parmesan
    cheese (optional)

> **Nutrition Tip:** Pizza can be made on many different crusts. You could increase your fiber by using whole wheat crust. You also save calories with thin crust versus thick crust or deep-dish pizzas. There are many other products you can use for a pizza treat, including pita or even English muffins. One benefit of using rice cakes or English muffins is portion control. If you serve one rice cake treat, your kids will be satisfied and learn early on what a proper portion is.
>
> Another idea is to make this a dessert pizza and top with cream cheese and assorted fresh fruits. What a fun way to introduce your child to star fruit, mandarin oranges, or kiwi!

1. Preheat oven to 325°F.
2. Place rice cakes on baking sheet. Spread 1 tablespoon of pizza sauce on each rice cake. Sprinkle ¼ cup grated mozzarella cheese on each cake. Sprinkle lightly with Parmesan cheese, if desired.
3. Bake until cheese melts, about 2 to 3 minutes.

Serving size: 1 cake; serves 8

Calories: 121
Carbohydrate: 11 grams
Protein: 8 grams
Fat: 5 grams

Fiber: 0 grams
Sodium: 220 milligrams
Cholesterol: 16 milligrams

15

• • •

Breads

Garlic Bread

2 cloves garlic, minced
2 teaspoons olive oil
2 teaspoons dried parsley
2 teaspoons dried thyme
¾ teaspoon dried marjoram

½ teaspoon paprika
2 tablespoons grated Parmesan
cheese
2 small (4-ounce) loaves Italian or
French bread

1. Preheat oven to 350°F.
2. Combine garlic and olive oil in a small bowl. Mix well.
3. Combine parsley, thyme, marjoram, and paprika in another small bowl. Add Parmesan cheese and mix well.
4. Cut each loaf of bread crosswise into diagonal slices without cutting all the way through. Brush cut sides of slices with garlic oil. Sprinkle herb mixture between slices.
5. Wrap each loaf in foil. Place on a baking sheet. Bake until heated through, about 10–15 minutes.

Serving size: 1 slice; serves 8

Calories: 65
Carbohydrate: 12 grams
Protein: 2 grams
Fat: 1 gram

Fiber: 1 gram
Sodium: 139 milligrams
Cholesterol: 0 milligrams

Nutrition Tip: Confused about fats and oils? All fats and oils add the same amount of calories: 9 calories per gram. Compare that to the calories from carbohydrates and proteins: 4 calories per gram. For this reason, fat is the first thing you want to monitor when watching your weight.

However, you can't and shouldn't eliminate all fats from your diet. The next step is to look at the type of fat. Mono- or polyunsaturated fats are better for you than saturated or trans fats. Olive oil as well as canola or varieties of nut oils are monounsaturated fats. Monounsaturated fats may help lower blood cholesterol levels but only if you are following a healthy diet plan overall.

Banana Bread

2 cups flour
1½ teaspoons baking powder
½ teaspoon baking soda
½ teaspoon salt
2 (4-ounce) cartons nonfat
    yogurt (any flavor)
1 cup mashed ripe banana
    (2-3 bananas)

½ cup sugar
¼ cup margarine, melted
2 eggs
1 teaspoon vanilla
    extract
vegetable cooking spray
2 teaspoons flour

1. Preheat oven to 350°F.
2. Combine flour, baking powder, baking soda, and salt in a large bowl. Make a well in center of mixture.
3. Combine yogurt, bananas, sugar, margarine, eggs, and vanilla extract. Add to dry ingredients. Stir just until dry ingredients are moistened.
4. Coat a loaf pan with cooking spray. Sprinkle with flour. Spoon batter into prepared pan. Bake for 1 hour, or until a wooden pick inserted in center comes out clean.
5. Let cool in pan 10 minutes. Remove from pan and let cool completely on a wire rack. Cut into 18 slices.

Serving size: one ½" slice

Calories: 123
Carbohydrate: 21 grams
Protein: 3 grams
Fat: 3 grams

Fiber: 1 gram
Sodium: 188 milligrams
Cholesterol: 24 milligrams

Nutrition Tip: This is a good way to use up overripe bananas as well as using the natural flavor of the bananas for the bread's sweetness. When making a quick bread, look for recipes that do not use a lot of sugar, or use sugar substitutes. A sugar substitute can significantly reduce the calories in a recipe, and there are many new products coming on the market that work well in baked foods. Read the manufacturer's recommendations for recipe substitutes.

Want to teach portion size? Make individual muffins instead of a loaf. Just pour the batter in a muffin tin, using cupcake liners if you like. You will reduce the cooking time, so watch carefully. One portion is a 2" muffin.

Jungle Bread

1½ cups flour
1 cup quick-cooking oats
¼ cup sugar
1 teaspoon baking powder
1 teaspoon baking soda
1 teaspoon cinnamon
½ teaspoon salt
1 teaspoon coconut extract
(optional)

¾ cup mashed, ripe bananas
(about 2 medium
bananas)
1 (8-ounce) can crushed
pineapple, with juice
¼ cup reduced-calorie
margarine, melted
2 eggs
Nonstick cooking spray

1. Preheat oven to 350°F.
2. Combine flour, oats, sugar, baking powder, baking soda, cinnamon, and salt in a large bowl.
3. Mix together coconut extract, banana, pineapple, margarine, and eggs in a medium bowl.
4. Add banana mixture to flour mixture. Stir just until liquid is absorbed and dry ingredients are thoroughly moistened. Do not overmix.
5. Coat a loaf pan with nonstick cooking spray. Pour mixture into pan. Bake for 50–55 minutes, or until wooden pick inserted in center comes out clean.
6. Cool in pan for 5 minutes. Loosen edges with knife and turn out onto cooling rack. Cool completely. Cut into 18 slices.

Nutrition Tip: Why is this called Jungle Bread? Coconuts, bananas, and pineapples can be found in a tropical jungle. What a fun way to introduce new fruits to your child. Try a snack of this bread while reading *The Jungle Book* together!

Another nutrition benefit from this recipe comes from the oatmeal. Oatmeal contains soluble fiber, which can help remove cholesterol from your body. Eating food rich in fiber helps to provide a sense of fullness and helps you feel full longer.

Serving size: one ½" slice

Calories: 106

Carbohydrate: 19 grams

Protein: 3 grams

Fat: 2 grams

Fiber: 1 gram

Sodium: 203 milligrams

Cholesterol: 24 milligrams

Focaccia

1 cup warm water (about 85°F)

1 package active, dry yeast

1 teaspoon sugar

⅓ cup olive oil (extravirgin best)

½ teaspoon salt

4 cups all-purpose flour, or 1 cup whole wheat flour

1 tablespoon fresh rosemary

1 teaspoon salt

¼ cup grated Parmesan cheese

1. Dissolve yeast in warm water and let sit for 5 minutes. Add sugar, oil, and salt. Mix until incorporated.
2. Add 1 cup of flour at a time. Use mixer with dough hook 3–4 minutes until thoroughly combined, or place dough on floured board and knead until dough is smooth and elastic.
3. First rise: Place dough in a greased bowl, cover, and let rise in a warm place until doubled in size, about 1 hour.
4. Punch dough down and let rest for 5–10 minutes.
5. Shaping and second rise: Roll dough into a ball. Place on an oiled jellyroll pan or cookie sheet. Flatten with hands or use a rolling pin, to ½-inch thickness. Dough will be full of bubbles and may not completely cover pan. Lightly brush with olive oil. Cover and let rise in a warm place 35–45 minutes.

6. Sprinkle with rosemary, salt, and Parmesan cheese. Push fingers into the dough to make pockmark indentations all over surface.
7. Bake at 400°F for 20–30 minutes, or until brown on top.
8. Cut into 12 slices.

Serving size: 1 slice

Calories: 215
Carbohydrate: 33 grams
Protein: 5 grams
Fat: 7 grams

Fiber: 1 gram
Sodium: 290 milligrams
Cholesterol: 1 milligram

Homemade Pizza

SAUCE

1 (15-ounce) can tomato puree (Italian style)
1 large clove garlic, minced
½ teaspoon dried oregano

½ teaspoon dried basil, or 1 teaspoon chopped fresh leaves
1 small bay leaf
Pepper to taste

DOUGH

1 package active, dry yeast
¼ cup warm water
2½-3 cups unbleached all-purpose flour, or use 1½ to 2 cups all-purpose flour and 1 cup whole wheat flour

¼ teaspoon salt
1 cup water
5 tablespoons olive oil
2 tablespoons cornmeal (optional)

1. Preheat oven to 450°F.
2. Place all sauce ingredients in saucepan. Cover and simmer for 30 minutes, stirring periodically. Remove bay leaf.
3. Dissolve yeast in ¼ cup warm water.
4. Place 1½ cups flour and salt in mixing bowl. Add 1 cup water, 2 tablespoons olive oil, and yeast to flour mixture. Mix with wooden spoon until all flour is incorporated. Slowly add remaining flour and mix until dough holds together.
5. Place dough on a well-floured board and knead until smooth and elastic, about 5 minutes. If dough becomes sticky, sprinkle a small amount of flour over it and continue to knead.
6. Place dough in a greased bowl, cover, and let rise in a warm place until doubled in size, about 1 hour.
7. Place on a lightly floured board. Punch dough down and let rest for 10–15 minutes.
8. Dough is ready to be divided, shaped, and topped (see table).
9. Brush pan lightly with part of the remaining oil and sprinkle with cornmeal. Bake for 15–20 minutes, or until crust is golden brown. Remove from oven and brush edge of crust with the rest of the olive oil.

Dough	Sauce	Grated Cheese	Cooked Meat	Vegetables	Servings
14" round	¾ cup	2 cups	1–2 cups	1–2 cups	8
Two 10" round	½ cup each	1 cup each	½–1 cup each	½–1 cup each	4 each
11"×16"	1 cup	2 cups	1–2 cups	1–2 cups	8+

Calories: 246   Fiber: 2 grams
Carbohydrate: 37 grams   Sodium: 287 milligrams
Protein: 5 grams   Cholesterol: 0 milligrams
Fat: 9 grams

Nutrition Tip: Homemade pizza sauce is great, but there are also many good commercial sauces. Be sure to check the fat content and choose the lower-fat varieties.

16

• • •

Fruity Treats

Fruit Yogurt Pops

1 (6-ounce) can frozen apple
juice concentrate
(or other juice), thawed
4 (4-ounce) containers
fat-free strawberry yogurt
(or other fruit)

10 (3-ounce) disposable
drinking cups
(or popsicle mold)
10 flat wooden sticks
(unless using popsicle mold)

1. Place drinking cups in square cake pan.
2. Place apple juice and yogurt in large liquid measuring cup or small pitcher. Stir until mixed well.
3. Pour mixture into cups until each cup is a little more than half full.
4. Place pan in freezer for 1 hour or until frozen enough for wooden sticks to stand up. Place one wooden stick in center of each pop. Freeze pops until completely frozen, about 4 hours.
5. Remove cups from pops and serve.

Serving size: 1 pop; serves 10

Calories: 52
Carbohydrate: 1 gram
Protein: 2 grams
Fat: 0 grams

Fiber: 0 grams
Sodium: 32 milligrams
Cholesterol: 0 milligrams

Orange Julius

¼ cup sugar
1 (6-ounce) can frozen
    orange juice concentrate,
    thawed

1 cup fat-free milk
1 cup water
1 teaspoon vanilla extract
10 ice cubes

In blender, combine all ingredients. Blend until ice cubes are crushed and beverage is smooth.

Serving size: 6 ounces; serves 4

Calories: 136
Carbohydrate: 31 grams
Protein: 3 grams
Fat: 1 gram

Fiber: 1 gram
Sodium: 35 milligrams
Cholesterol: 1 milligram

APPENDIX A: FORMS

• • •

- Family Assessment Tool
- Family Goals
- Daily Food Record
- MyPyramid

FAMILY ASSESSMENT TOOL

	Sun	Mon	Tues	Wed	Thurs	Fri	Sat
1. How many hours per day does my child watch TV, play video or computer games?							
2. How many times per day do you drink soda or sweet drinks (including sports drinks)?							
3. How many hours do you exercise or have active playtime?							
4. How many times does the family eat out?							
5. How many times do you eat together as a family?							
6. How many servings of fruit and vegetables do you eat each day?							
7. Do you prepare meals and snacks that you plan for the day?							

NOTES:

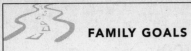

FAMILY GOALS

	Family	Adults	Child 1	Child 2
Parenting Goal				
Specific goal:				
Measure:				
Time frame:				
Healthy Behaviors Goal				
Specific goal:				
Measure:				
Time frame:				
Healthy Food Goal				
Specific goal:				
Measure:				
Time frame:				
Fitness Goal				
Specific goal:				
Measure:				
Time frame:				

NOTES:

DAILY FOOD RECORD

Name: _____ Date: _____

Circle Day: MON   TUE   WED   THUR   FRI   SAT   SUN

	What I Ate	How Much I Ate
Breakfast		
Morning Snack		
Lunch		
Afternoon Snack		
Dinner		
Evening Snack		

Exercise Completed

MyPyramid:
How Does Your Pyramid Stack Up?

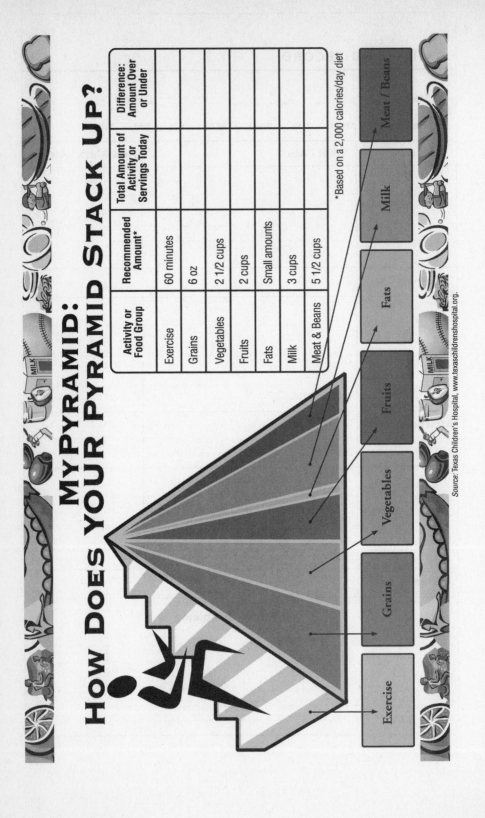

Activity or Food Group	Recommended Amount*	Total Amount of Activity or Servings Today	Difference: Amount Over or Under
Exercise	60 minutes		
Grains	6 oz		
Vegetables	2 1/2 cups		
Fruits	2 cups		
Fats	Small amounts		
Milk	3 cups		
Meat & Beans	5 1/2 cups		

*Based on a 2,000 calories/day diet

Exercise Grains Vegetables Fruits Fats Milk Meat / Beans

Source: Texas Children's Hospital, www.texaschildrenshospital.org.

APPENDIX B: TOOLS

. . .

- Food Quiz
- Low-Fat Recipe Substitutions
- Food Group Portion Sizes
- Healthy Shopping List
- Can You See Obesity? Calculating Body Mass Index

Food Quiz

Hey, kids! Did you know that having the right info about food can help you make smart choices? Take this quiz—and find out what you know and don't know. You might be surprised!

1. Oatmeal is part of which food group?
   a. Dairy
   b. Fruit
   c. Grains

2. Ice cream belongs with which food group?
   a. Dairy
   b. Fats and others
   c. Meat, beans, and protein

3. Eggs belong with which food group?
   a. Vegetables
   b. Meat and proteins
   c. Dairy

4. Which food is lowest in fat and is the healthiest food choice?
   a. Grilled chicken with no skin
   b. Baked chicken with skin
   c. Fried chicken

5. Fat-free foods mean I can eat more than the regular version.
   True or False

6. Juice is good for me and I should drink 2 cups a day.
   True or False

7. Regular soda is calorie free.
   True or False

8. Fiber helps keep food moving through the body. Foods in which group have the most fiber in them?
   a. Meat and proteins
   b. Fats and others
   c. Fruits and vegetables

9. Which of the following makes the healthiest snack?
   a. 3 cookies and low-fat milk
   b. 1 small bag of potato chips and soda
   c. 3 celery sticks with peanut butter and 1 cup of low-fat milk

10. How many different food groups are in MyPyramid?
    a. 4—Meat, Vegetables, Protein, Bread
    b. 5—Meat, Vegetables, Fruit, Dairy, Grains
    c. 6—Meat/Protein, Vegetables, Fruit, Dairy, Grains, Fats and others

11. The jelly portion of a Pop-T art is considered a fruit serving.
    True or False

12. An individual-size bottle of juice is considered one serving.
    True or False

Answers to Food Quiz

1. C—Grains. Oatmeal is made from oats, which are a type of grain grown in a field.
2. B—Fats and others. Although ice cream is made from milk, it has a lot of fat in it, so it belongs in the Fats and others category. Tricky!
3. B—Meat and proteins group. Eggs are an animal protein and chock-full of protein to make muscles grow strong.
4. A—Grilled chicken with no skin. Fried chicken not only has the skin on it but also is cooked in hot oil, which has extra fat that adds calories to the meat. Baked chicken with the skin is lower in fat than fried chicken but is still higher in fat because the skin is fatty.
5. False—Just because the label says "fat free" does not mean the food is calorie free. It is the overall calorie amount you eat each day balanced with the calories you burn that affect weight gain or weight loss.
6. False—Although juice is made from whole fruits, it contains large amounts of sugar. The extra sugar adds up to extra calories that your body does not need.
7. False—Regular soda usually contains about 150 calories per 12 ounces. Diet soda usually contains no or very low amounts of calories.
8. C—Fruits and vegetables. These two groups of food are plants, which is where fiber comes from. The fiber they provide helps keep us "regular" when going to the bathroom.
9. C—A good, filling snack usually consists of foods from at least two of the major groups. This example has celery (vegetable), peanut butter (meat and protein), and low-fat milk (dairy). The other two snacks include foods from the Fats and others category—cookies, potato chips, and soda.
10. C—MyPyramid has six different food groups:
    Grains
    Vegetables
    Fruit
    Fats and others
    Dairy
    Meat/Protein
11. False—There is very little fruit in the center and too much sugar for a Pop-Tart to be considered a fruit serving.
12. False—Be careful. For juice to be considered a fruit serving, it must be 100 percent fruit juice. Also, one serving is 4 ounces. If your bottle is more than 4 ounces, and most are, you have multiple servings. Remember not to drink too many of your calories! Fill up on healthy foods.

Low-Fat Recipe Substitutions

Here are a few adjustments you can make to your favorite recipes to minimize the fat content in your daily diet.

If Recipe Calls For	Use or Substitute
Bacon	• Turkey bacon
Beef, ground	• Ground turkey • Extralean ground beef • Vegetarian meat (textured vegetable protein)
Butter or oil for baking and cooking	• Low-fat margarine • Nonfat margarine • Applesauce • Pureed fruits • Pureed vegetables 1 cup .(fat=⅔ cup fruit substitute)
Butter for browning	• Nonstick spray* • Chicken broth • Beef broth • Wine • Water-oil spray
Cheese	• Low-fat cheese • A smaller amount of a "sharp" cheese
Chicken	• White-meat chicken, skinned • Turkey breast, skinned
Cottage cheese	• Low-fat cottage cheese • Nonfat cottage cheese
Cream, heavy (used in recipes, not for whipping)	• Fat-free half-and-half • 2 tablespoons flour whisked into 2 cups nonfat milk • Fat-free evaporated milk

(continued)

(continued)

If Recipe Calls For	Use or Substitute
Cream, whipping	• Evaporated skim milk, chilled
Cream cheese	• Low-fat cream cheese • Nonfat cream cheese • Low-fat or nonfat yogurt cheese
Creamed soup	• Low-fat creamed soup
Eggs	• 2 egg whites for each egg • Egg substitute
Mayonnaise	• Low-fat mayonnaise • Nonfat mayonnaise
Whole milk or buttermilk	• 2% milk • Skim milk • Low-fat or nonfat buttermilk
Peanut butter	• Natural or reduced-fat peanut butter
Pork	• Turkey ham • Lean cuts
Sour cream	• Low-fat sour cream • Nonfat sour cream • Low-fat yogurt • Nonfat yogurt • Blend 1 cup of low-fat cottage cheese with skim milk and lemon juice to taste
Tuna	• Tuna packed in water
Vegetable oil (in salad dressing or marinade)	• Wine • Broth

*Make your own nonstick spray by filling a spray bottle ⅔ full with water and the remaining ⅓ with your favorite cooking oil. This can be sprayed in pans or directly on food for a light coating of oil.

FOOD GROUP PORTION SIZES

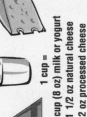
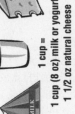

MILK

1 cup =
1 cup (8 oz) milk or yogurt
1 1/2 oz natural cheese
2 oz processed cheese

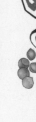
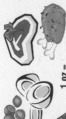

MEAT/BEANS

1 oz =
1 oz meat, poultry, or fish
1/4 cup cooked, dry beans
1 tablespoon peanut butter
1/4 cup nuts or seeds
1 egg

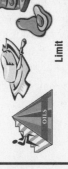

OILS

Limit
Oil   Butter/margarine
Mayonnaise   Olives
Peanut butter   Nuts
Salad dressing   Avocado

---

1 1/2 oz of cheese is about the size of six stacked dice.

3 oz of meat is about the size of a deck of playing cards.

1 teaspoon of peanut butter is about the size of the tip of your thumb.

STAY PHYSICALLY ACTIVE

PHYSICAL

Physical activity is any movement of the body that uses energy, like walking, climbing the stairs, swimming, playing basketball, or dancing.

Children & teenagers should participate in moderate or vigorous physical activity for 60 minutes every day.

FOOD GROUP PORTION SIZES

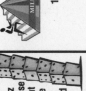
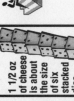

GRAINS

1 oz =
1 slice of bread
1 cup ready-to-eat cereal
1/2 cup cooked rice, pasta, cereal

1/2 cup of cooked pasta is about the size of a tennis ball.

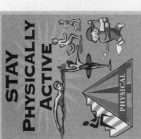

VEGETABLES

1 cup =
1 cup raw or cooked vegetables
1 cup (8 oz) vegetable juice
2 cups raw leafy greens

1 cup of vegetables is about the size of your fist.

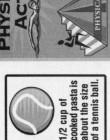

FRUITS

1 cup =
1 cup fresh fruit
1 cup (8 oz) 100% fruit juice
1/2 cup dried fruit

1 cup of fruit is about the size of a baseball.

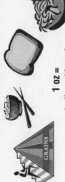

Source: Texas Children's Hospital, www.texaschildrenshospital.org.

Healthy Shopping List

This list suggests healthy choices to make at the grocery store. There may be items in the Healthy Items column that your family will not eat and items in the Limit or Avoid column that are your family's favorite items. Try for a balance of healthy choices—about eight out of ten items in your grocery cart should be healthy. That leaves you about two of every ten limit or avoid items to meet your family's food preferences. A good example is breakfast cereal. If your children want only one brand of high-sugar cereal, it may be okay if the cereal is eaten with skim milk and fresh fruit and the rest of the grains in their diet are whole grain.

HEALTHY ITEMS	LIMIT OR AVOID
Milk and Dairy	
Low-fat or skim milk	Whole milk
Low-fat cheese: ricotta, mozzarella	High-fat cheese
Nonfat or low-fat yogurt	Cream
Meat and Protein Sources	
Beef—chuck, 90% lean ground beef, round steak or roast, rump roast	Beef and pork with visible fat
	Ground beef with more than 10% fat
Pork—Canadian bacon; well-trimmed ham; loin rib, chop, or roast	Sausage
	Regular hot dogs
Fish or shellfish—all, fresh or frozen, unbreaded; canned tuna or salmon in water	High-fat luncheon meats like bologna
	Ribs
Poultry—chicken or turkey, all skin removed	Fried fish or shellfish
	Fried chicken
Luncheon meats—97% or higher fat-free sliced meats or hot dogs	Chicken or turkey with skin
	Limit processed nut butters
Eggs—whites are unlimited, but limit yolks, egg substitutes	
Nut butters—natural peanut, almond, or cashew reduced-fat peanut butter	
Breads, Cereals, Grains	
100% whole wheat sliced breads, buns, rolls	Biscuits

(continued)

HEALTHY ITEMS	LIMIT OR AVOID
Reduced-fat whole-grain crackers, graham crackers	Croissants
Wheat, corn, oat, or other whole-grain cereals with low added sugar	Doughnuts
	Sweet rolls
	Presweetened cereals
	Regular chips—potato, corn
Whole wheat—spaghetti, macaroni, noodles	High-fat crackers
Brown rice or rice cakes	Regular pasta and white rice
Air-popped popcorn	Fried rice
Corn tortillas	Flour tortillas

Vegetables

All fresh vegetables	Vegetables with added fat like bacon, cream sauces, or cheese
All canned or frozen vegetables except those with added fat or sauces	Fried vegetables
100% vegetable juices	

Starchy Vegetables

Sweet potatoes	Limit white potatoes, especially french fries
Winter squash	Creamed corn
Peas	Beans with added fat like ham or bacon
Dried beans, peas, lentils	

Fruits and Juices

All fresh fruits	Fruit pies
Canned fruits in juice	Canned fruit in syrup
100% fruit juice	Sweetened or artificial juice drinks

Desserts (in moderation)

Angel food cake	Cake or cupcakes
Ice milk	Ice cream
Low-fat frozen yogurt	Cookies
Pudding made with skim milk	Pies
Reduced-fat cookies	

Fats

Oil—canola, corn, cottonseed, olive, soybean	Butter
	Bacon
Margarine—soft tub or liquid margarine	Cream
	Lard or shortening

(continued)

HEALTHY ITEMS	LIMIT OR AVOID
Salad dressing—"lite" or fat free	Hard margarine
Reduced-fat mayonnaise	Regular salad dressings

Miscellaneous

Jelly and jams—100% fruit spreads	Jelly
Mustard	Honey
Ketchup	Sugar
Salsa	
Spices and herbs	

Can You See Obesity?
Calculating Body Mass Index

Body Mass Index (BMI) is more realistic than weight as a measure of health. BMI for age correlates with clinical risk factors for cardiovascular disease, elevated insulin levels, and high blood pressure. The calculation is based on a combination of height and weight.

The terms *at risk for overweight, overweight,* and *obese* are defined and measured differently for adults and for children. Although the method of calculation is the same, the standards are based on age and therefore differ. For adults, thresholds can help determine the degree of overweight.

Instead of set thresholds for underweight and overweight for children, the BMI percentile is what is important in children two to twenty years of age. For children, BMI is gender and age specific. A BMI that is less than the 5th percentile is underweight and one that is above the 95th percentile is overweight. Children with a BMI between the 85th and 95th percentile are considered at risk of becoming overweight. Find the BMI charts in Appendix C or use the CDC Web site BMI calculator at www.cdc.gov/nccdphp/dnpa/bmi/index.htm.

Calculating BMI Using Pounds and Inches

When using pounds and inches to calculate BMI, ounces and fractions must be changed to decimal values. For example 36½ pounds becomes 36.5 pounds. To calculate BMI, divide the weight in pounds by the height in inches squared, then multiply by 703.

$$BMI = \frac{\text{weight in pounds}}{(\text{height in inches}) \times (\text{height in inches})} \times 703$$

Example: Calculating BMI

Joshua is four years old. His weight is 47 pounds 4 ounces. His height is 41½ inches.

Step 1. Joshua's weight of 47 pounds and 4 oz = 47.25 pounds

Step 2. Joshua's height of 41½ inches = 41.5 inches

Step 3. Calculate: $\frac{47.25}{41.5 \times 41.5} \times 703 = 19.2$

Step 4. Look at the BMI chart for boys 2 to 20 years old. Joshua is overweight because his BMI is greater than the 95th percentile.

BMI Categories for Adults

Normal weight	=	18.5 to 24.9
Overweight	=	25.0 to 29.9
Obese, Class I	=	30.0 to 34.9
Obese, Class II	=	35.0 to 39.9
Obese, Class III	=	40.0 and up

BMI Categories for Children

Underweight=below 5th percentile
Normal=between 5th and 85th percentile
At risk of overweight=between 85th and 95th percentile
Overweight=greater than 95th percentile

APPENDIX C: GROWTH CHARTS

2 to 20 years: Boys
Body mass index-for-age percentiles

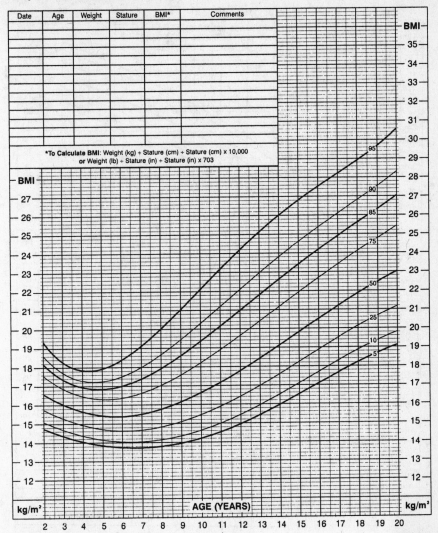

Date	Age	Weight	Stature	BMI*	Comments

*To Calculate BMI: Weight (kg) ÷ Stature (cm) ÷ Stature (cm) x 10,000
or Weight (lb) ÷ Stature (in) ÷ Stature (in) x 703

BMI

AGE (YEARS)

kg/m²

kg/m²

Published May 30, 2000 (modified 10/16/00).
SOURCE: Developed by the National Center for Health Statistics in collaboration with
the National Center for Chronic Disease Prevention and Health Promotion (2000).
http://www.cdc.gov/growthcharts

SAFER · HEALTHIER · PEOPLE™

Birth to 36 months: Boys
Length-for-age and Weight-for-age percentiles

NAME _____

RECORD # _____

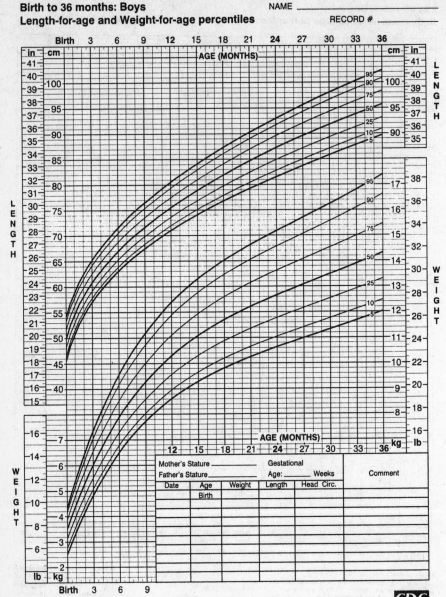

Published May 30, 2000 (modified 4/20/01).
SOURCE: Developed by the National Center for Health Statistics in collaboration with
the National Center for Chronic Disease Prevention and Health Promotion (2000).
http://www.cdc.gov/growthcharts

SAFER · HEALTHIER · PEOPLE™

Birth to 36 months: Boys
Head circumference-for-age and
Weight-for-length percentiles

NAME _____

RECORD # _____

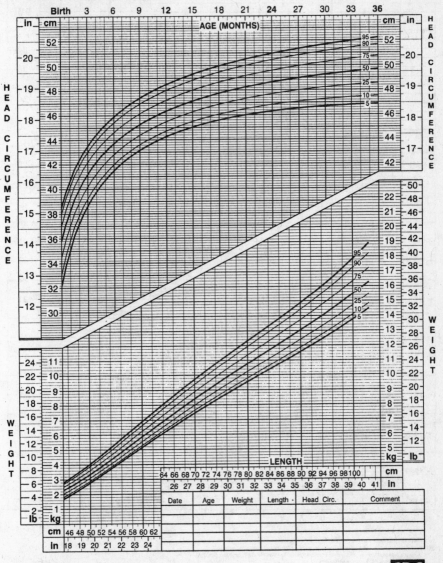

Published May 30, 2000 (modified 10/16/00).
SOURCE: Developed by the National Center for Health Statistics in collaboration with
the National Center for Chronic Disease Prevention and Health Promotion (2000).
http://www.cdc.gov/growthcharts

2 to 20 years: Girls
Body mass index-for-age percentiles

NAME _____

RECORD # _____

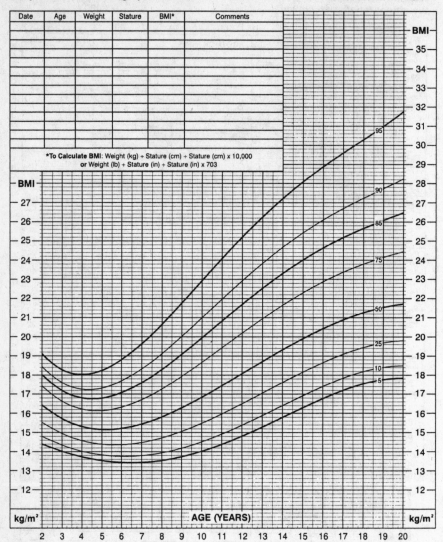

Date	Age	Weight	Stature	BMI*	Comments

*To Calculate BMI: Weight (kg) ÷ Stature (cm) ÷ Stature (cm) x 10,000
or Weight (lb) ÷ Stature (in) ÷ Stature (in) x 703

AGE (YEARS)

Published May 30, 2000 (modified 10/16/00).
SOURCE: Developed by the National Center for Health Statistics in collaboration with
the National Center for Chronic Disease Prevention and Health Promotion (2000).
http://www.cdc.gov/growthcharts

Birth to 36 months: Girls
Length-for-age and Weight-for-age percentiles

NAME _____

RECORD # _____

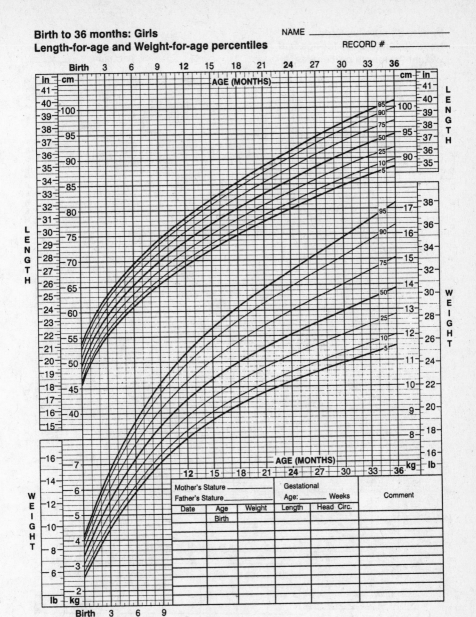

Published May 30, 2000 (modified 4/20/01).
SOURCE: Developed by the National Center for Health Statistics in collaboration with
the National Center for Chronic Disease Prevention and Health Promotion (2000).
http://www.cdc.gov/growthcharts

Birth to 36 months: Girls
Head circumference-for-age and
Weight-for-length percentiles

NAME _____

RECORD # _____

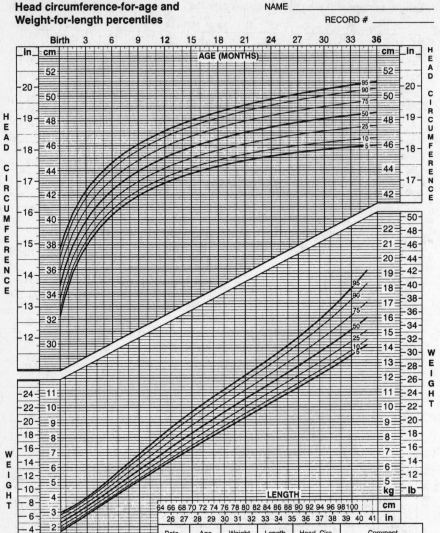

Published May 30, 2000 (modified 10/16/00).
SOURCE: Developed by the National Center for Health Statistics in collaboration with
the National Center for Chronic Disease Prevention and Health Promotion (2000).
http://www.cdc.gov/growthcharts

Nutrition Glossary

amino acids. Building blocks that make protein.

antioxidants. Substances that suppress oxygen reactions.

carbohydrates. Carbohydrates are sugars, fibers, and starches that are basically chains of sugar molecules. Carbohydrates are classified as *simple sugars* and *complex carbohydrates*. Simple sugars, such as glucose and fructose, are carbohydrates in their simplest form and do not need to be broken down in the body before being absorbed into the bloodstream. Simple sugars like sucrose, or table sugar, and lactose are made of two sugar molecules, while the more complex carbohydrates like starches, such as those found in grains, root vegetables, and legumes, are made up of hundreds of sugar molecules. *Fiber,* a type of carbohydrate that cannot be digested in the human digestive tract, is in all plant foods, including grains, beans, vegetables, and fruits. Eating enough fiber can have beneficial effects on the risk factors for heart disease, blood sugar control, and constipation.

fats and fatty acids. Fats are chains of fatty acids. Simply, fats are substances that do not dissolve in water and can be digested. Fats are required by the body for support of body structures and absorption of fat-soluble vitamins—A, D, E, and K. Fats also supply energy. Every gram of fat supplies 9 calories of energy, more than twice as much as carbohydrates or proteins. *Saturated fats* come primarily from animal sources, although coconut and palm oils also are saturated. *Unsaturated fats* come from vegetables, nuts, and seeds. Unsaturated fats are the "good" fats because they help lower cholesterol in the blood. The two main types of unsaturated fats are polyunsaturated and monounsaturated. Polyunsaturated fats are in sunflower, corn, and soybean oils; monounsaturated fats are in canola, peanut, and olive oils. *Omega-3 fatty acids* are another type of unsaturated fat, found primarily in fatty fish, such as salmon or sardines. This fatty acid may have a beneficial effect on heart disease by protecting the heart from rhythm disturbances. The American Heart Association recommends eating two servings of fish each week. Unsaturated fats can be made more saturated by adding hydrogen, which produces a harder, more stable fat. It also produces *trans fats,* such as those found in processed foods and stick margarines. Saturated and trans fats are the "bad" fats that boost the level of cholesterol in the blood.

free radicals. Charged compounds that react with chemicals in the body.

metabolism. A chemical process in living things that distributes nutrients and provides energy from food.

minerals. Nonliving substances that occur in nature. They are compounds that may contain metals, nonmetals, ions, or phosphates. Minerals are important for many body functions including water balance, use of energy, and transmission of genetic information. Minerals must be obtained from food to prevent deficiencies.

Iron is an essential mineral that is found in every cell of the body. It is found in a protein called hemoglobin in the blood and myoglobin in muscle cells. These proteins bind to oxygen and carry it from the lungs to the cells to be used. Iron is also found in many body proteins and enzymes.

Phosphorus is a mineral that is found primarily in bones and teeth. In addition to forming bones and teeth, phosphorus is important in digestion of carbohydrates and fat. It is important in the use of protein for growth and maintenance of body tissues. It assists proper functioning of the muscles, kidneys, heart, and nervous system.

Magnesium is a mineral that is essential for the production and use of energy. It helps muscles contract and relax, helps form protein, and assists enzymes in the body.

Potassium is a mineral that is important for proper functioning of cells and electrical activity in the body. Potassium assists in water balance, making proteins, using carbohydrates, building muscle, and proper functioning of nerves and the brain.

Sodium helps regulate blood pressure and blood volume. It is also used for normal functioning of muscles and nerves.

Chloride helps maintain the proper acidity of the blood and is part of the digestive juices in the stomach. Chloride is found in table salt and in foods such as tomatoes, lettuce, celery, and olives.

mucous membrane. Tissues that line parts of the body that open to the outside, such as the nose, mouth, and digestive tract.

protein. Protein performs many functions that are essential for life: growth and repair of body tissues; balance of fluid, enzymes, and hormones; and fighting infection. Proteins are made up of amino acids. The amino acids form chains that develop into the many different structures and chemicals needed by the body.

sugar substitutes. *Saccharin* is the oldest of the currently approved sweeteners. It is a derivative of coal tar and is 300 times sweeter than sugar. The body does not digest it, so it is calorie free. The use of saccharin has significantly decreased because studies linked it to bladder cancer in mice. It is still used in diet soft drinks, baked goods, and as a powdered sweetener, usually sold as Sweet 'n Low.

Aspartame is made by combining two amino acids found naturally in protein foods. It is 200 times sweeter than sugar and is digested just like any other protein but is virtually calorie free. Aspartame loses its sweetness in high heat, so can be difficult to use in cooking. It is used frequently in soft drinks, frozen desserts, and puddings, and as a powdered sweetener with the brand names NutraSweet and Equal. Aspartame cannot be used by people with phenylketonuria (PKU), which is a metabolic disorder that causes the accumulation of amino acid phenylalanine in the body.

Acesulfame-K is similar to saccharine. It is 150 to 200 times sweeter than sugar. The body does not digest it, so it is calorie free. It is used in baked goods, desserts, syrups, candies, and yogurt, and as a powdered sweetener with the brand names Sunette, Sweet One, and Sweet 'n Safe.

Sucralose is made by adding chloride to a sugarlike molecule. It is 600 times sweeter than sugar. The body does not digest it, so it is calorie free. It is used in baked goods, sodas, gum, and candies, and as a powdered sweetener with the brand name Splenda.

Tagatose is a new sweetener made by changing the structure of milk sugar. It is not digested by the body so it is calorie free. It is not yet used in many products, except for some beverages, but eventually may be used in cereals, yogurt, ice cream, candy, and gum, and as a powdered sweetener with the brand name Naturlose.

Sugar alcohols are made by adding hydrogen to sugar molecules. They do not contain ethanol so are not related in any way to alcoholic beverages. There are many different types of sugar alcohols: *sorbitol, xylitol, malitol,* and others. Some have almost as many calories as sugar; others are not well digested and have almost no calories. Sugar alcohols are found in many "sugar-free" foods such as candy, cookies, chewing gum, and soft drinks. They are also found in toothpaste, mouthwash, and throat lozenges. Eating too many sugar alcohols can have a laxative effect, causing bloating, gas, and diarrhea.

vitamins. Nutrients that your body needs in very small quantities, called *micronutrients,* for normal functioning. They must be obtained from food because they cannot be made in the body. Four of the vitamins are fat soluble and can accumulate in the body: A, D, E, and K. The others are water soluble and any excess is excreted: B_1, B_2, B_6, B_{12}, C, biotin, folic acid, pantothenic acid, and niacin.

Vitamin A is used to form healthy skin, hair, and mucous membranes, and is necessary for proper bone growth, tooth development, eyesight, and reproduction. Vitamin A is found in fortified cereals and dairy products as well as in fruits and vegetables.

Vitamin D primarily maintains normal blood levels of calcium and phosphorus. It aids in the absorption of calcium, helping to form and maintain strong bones. Vitamin D is found in enriched dairy products, fish, and eggs. The sun is also an important source of vitamin D, which forms on the skin. Ten minutes a day in the sun can form enough vitamin D to meet your normal needs.

Vitamin E is an antioxidant that helps protect cells from damage by free radicals, which are potentially damaging by-products of energy metabolism. Vitamin E is found in enriched grains such as enriched breakfast cereals, fruits, green leafy vegetables, fish, nuts, seeds, and vegetable oils.

Vitamin K is required for normal blood clotting. It is used in the liver to make the factors that help blood to clot. Vitamin K is found in green leafy vegetables, meats, grains, and dairy products. Vitamin K is also made in the large intestine by normal bacteria found in the gut.

Vitamin B_1 is also known as thiamin. It is important in helping the body release energy from carbohydrates and for proper nervous system functioning. Thiamin is available in most enriched grain products such as breakfast cereal, melons, orange juice, meats (especially pork), corn, and peas.

Vitamin B_2, or riboflavin, is essential for the release of energy from carbohydrates, fats, and protein in the diet. Riboflavin is available in enriched grain products such as breakfast cereal, broccoli, mushrooms, spinach, sweet potatoes, lean meats, and low-fat dairy products.

Vitamin B_6, also called pyridoxine, is used by the body to help build tissues from protein and metabolize fat. Increasing protein in the diet increases the need for vitamin B_6. Pyridoxine is found in enriched grains such as breakfast cereals, bananas, watermelon, potatoes, spinach, tomatoes, lean meats, poultry, and fish, including salmon.

Vitamin B_{12}, or cobalamin, is used to form red blood cells, maintain nervous system functioning, and metabolize protein and fat. Vitamin B_{12} is found only in animal foods: meat, poultry, fish, and dairy products.

Vitamin C, also known as ascorbic acid, is needed to form collagen, a building block for body structures such as bones, muscles, cartilage, and blood vessels. Vitamin C also helps the body absorb iron from food. The best sources of vitamin C are fruits and vegetables, especially citrus fruits such as oranges.

Biotin is necessary for formation of fatty acids and glucose, which are used to produce energy. It is also important for the metabolism of amino acids and carbohydrates. Biotin is made in the large intestine by normal bacteria found in the gut. It is also available in liver, cooked eggs, and yeast.

Folic acid is important to help the body form red blood cells. It reduces the incidence of nervous system defects in infants whose mothers eat enough folic acid while pregnant. Folic acid is found in enriched grains such as breakfast cereals, citrus fruits, poultry, many green vegetables, and dried beans and peas.

Pantothenic acid is essential for the metabolism of protein, fat, and carbohydrate, and for the body to make hormones and cholesterol. Good sources of pantothenic acid include enriched grains such as enriched breakfast cereals, lean beef, eggs, fish, dairy products, broccoli, and potatoes.

Niacin is necessary for a healthy digestive system, skin, and nerves and for the conversion of food to energy. Niacin is found in enriched grains such as enriched breakfast cereals, meat, poultry, fish, and eggs. Niacin can also be formed in the body.

Web Sites

www.dole5aday.com An interactive site for kids, parents, health professionals, and educators that helps to promote the importance of fruits and vegetables in our daily lives.

www.eatright.org American Dietetic Association's Web site, which features a daily nutrition tip, position papers on nutrition-related subjects, and a "search" button for easy information gathering.

www.fitday.com Designed to help you track and analyze the important aspects of your diet and fitness. Serves as a food and exercise journal. Based on your journal entry, the Web site analyzes your diet, exercise, and weight.

www.gatorade.com Information on sports nutrition and the importance of hydration. An interactive tour of how sports drinks work in your body.

www.health-fitness-tips.com A free weekly newsletter sent to your e-mail address offers tips for exercise and healthy living.

www.mardiweb.com/lowfat A forum for people interested in adopting a low-fat lifestyle. Features many recipes, tips for eating out, low-fat cooking strategies, facts about fast food, and more.

www.mypyramid.gov Features nutritional information for kids, parents, and professionals based on MyPyramid plan. Very interactive, with many handouts, posters, and brochures.

www.nationaldairycouncil.org An informative site developed to educate about the importance of dairy products. Offers nutrition and product information, resources, tools for schools, news, and recipes.

www.quackwatch.com Your guide to health fraud and quackery. Get information on questionable products, services, and theories (e.g., cellulite blockers, Atkins diet, and supplements).

www.tnp.com   The Natural Pharmacist is a science-based Web site that provides natural health information about supplements, herbs, drug interactions, alternative therapies, and medical conditions from allergies to heart failure. Click the "printer friendly" button for easier reading.

www.weightloss.com   Describes the basics of weight loss. Assess your body mass index (BMI); take a diet persona quiz; learn tips for smart eating, cutting fat from food, exercise, and remaining positive.

www.weightwatchers.com   Read inspirational success stories of weight loss, weight-loss tips, and low-fat recipes. Includes a recipe of the day.

References

Abramovitz, B. A., and L. L. Birch. 2000. "Five-Year-Old Girls' Ideas About Dieting Are Predicted by Their Mothers' Dieting." *J Am Diet Assoc* 100 (10): 1157–63.

Academy of General Dentistry. "Early Childhood Tooth Decay: Is Your Child at Risk?" www.agd.org/consumer/topics/baby/sippycup.asp.

Addessi, E., A. T. Galloway, E. Visalberghi, and L. L. Birch. 2005. "Specific Social Influences on the Acceptance of Novel Foods in 2–5-Year-Old-Children." *Appetite* 45 (3): 264–71.

American Alliance for Health, Physical Education, Recreation & Dance. "NASPE Releases First Ever Physical Activity Guidelines for Infants & Toddlers." 2002. www.aahperd.org/NASPE/infantstoddlers.html.

American Dietetic Association 1999. "Nutrition Standards for Child-Care Programs." *J Am Diet Assoc* 99 (8): 981–88.

———. 2004. "Kids' Breakfast Pyramid: Featuring Kids' Top 25 Favorite Breakfast Picks." www.eatright.org/ada/files/nfs0103.pdf.

———. "Eating Better Together: A Family Guide for a Healthier Lifestyle." 2005. www.eatright.org/ada/files/0305_Factsheet_Wendys.pdf.

American Dietetic Association and WellPoint Health Networks. "Healthy Habits for Healthy Kids: A Nutrition and Activity Guide for Parents." 2003. www.eatright.org/ada/files/wellpoint.pdf.

American Heart Association. "Eating Out and About." www.americanheart.org/presenter.jhtml?identifier=531.

Armstrong, J., and J. J. Reilly. 2002. "Breastfeeding and Lowering the Risk of Childhood Obesity." *Lancet* 359 (9322): 2003–04.

Arnon, S. S. 1980. "Honey, Infant Botulism and the Sudden Infant Death Syndrome." *West J Med* 132 (1): 58–59.

Baker, J. L., K. F. Michaelsen, K. M. Rasmussen, and T. I. Sorensen. 2004. "Maternal Prepregnant Body Mass Index, Duration of Breastfeeding, and Timing of Complementary Food Introduction Are Associated with Infant Weight Gain." *Am J Clin Nutr* 80 (6): 579–88.

Basciano, H., L. Federico, and K. Adeli. 2005. "Fructose, Insulin Resistance, and Metabolic Dyslipidemia." *Nutr Metab (Lond)* 2 (1): 5.

Befort, C., H. Kaur, N. Nollen, D. K. Sullivan, N. Nazir, W. S. Choi, L. Hornberger, and J. S. Ahluwalia. 2006 "Fruit, Vegetable, and Fat Intake Among non-Hispanic Black and non-Hispanic White Adolescents: Associations with Home Availability and Food Consumption Settings." *J Am Diet Assoc* 106 (3): 367–73.

Berkey, C. S., H. R. Rockett, M. W. Gillman, A. E. Field, and G. A. Colditz. 2003. "Longitudinal Study of Skipping Breakfast and Weight Change in Adolescents." *Int J Obes Relat Metab Disord* 27 (10): 1258–66.

Bernhardt, D. T., J. Gomez, M. D. Johnson, T. J. Martin, T. W. Rowland, E. Small, C. LeBlanc, R. Malina, C. Krein, J. C. Young, F. E. Reed, S. J. Anderson, B. A. Griesemer, and O. Bar-Or. 2001. "Strength Training by Children and Adolescents." *Pediatrics* 107 (6): 1470–2.

Birch, L. L., and J. O. Fisher. 1998. "Development of Eating Behaviors Among Children and Adolescents." *Pediatrics* 101 (3 Pt 2): 539–49.

Bogen, D. L., B. H. Hanusa, and R. C. Whitaker. 2004. "The Effect of Breast-Feeding with and Without Formula Use on the Risk of Obesity at 4 Years of Age." *Obes Res* 12 (9): 1527–35.

Buchowski, M. S., K. M. Majchrzak, K. Blomquist, K. Y. Chen, D. W. Byrne, and J. A. Bachorowski. 2006. "Energy Expenditure of Genuine Laughter." *Int J Obes (Lond)* 31 (1): 131–37.

Campbell, K. J., D. A. Crawford, and K. Ball. 2006. "Family Food Environment and Dietary Behaviors Likely to Promote Fatness in 5–6 Year-Old Children." *Int J Obes (Lond)* 30 (8): 1272–80.

Carruth, B. R., and J. D. Skinner. 2002. "Feeding Behaviors and Other Motor Development in Healthy Children (2–24 Months)." *J Am Coll Nutr* 21 (2): 88–96.

Carruth, B. R., P. J. Ziegler, A. Gordon, and K. Hendricks. 2004. "Developmental Milestones and Self-Feeding Behaviors in Infants and Toddlers." *J Am Diet Assoc* 104 (1 Suppl 1): s51–56.

Case-Smith, J., and R. Humphry. 2005. "Feeding Intervention." In *Occupational Therapy for Children*, edited by J. Case-Smith. St. Louis: Mosby.

Cason, K. L. 2006. "Family Mealtimes: More than Just Eating Together." *J Am Diet Assoc* 106 (4): 532–33.

Channel One Network. 1998. *A Day in the Life of a Teen's Appetite*.

Cho, S., M. Dietrich, C. J. Brown, C. A. Clark, and G. Block. 2003. "The Effect of Breakfast Type on Total Daily Energy Intake and Body Mass Index: Results from the Third National Health and Nutrition Examination Survey (NHANES III)." *J Am Coll Nutr* 22 (4): 296–302.

Christakis, D. A., B. E. Ebel, F. P. Rivara, and F. J. Zimmerman. 2004. "Television, Video, and Computer Game Usage in Children Under 11 Years of Age." *J Pediatr* 145 (5): 652–56.

Cullen, K. W., T. Baranowski, E. Owens, T. Marsh, L. Rittenberry, and C. de Moor. 2003. "Availability, Accessibility, and Preferences for Fruit, 100% Fruit Juice, and Vegetables Influence Children's Dietary Behavior." *Health Educ Behav* 30 (5): 615–26.

Cummings, S., E. S. Parham, and G. W. Strain. 2002. "Position of the American Dietetic Association: Weight Management." *J Am Diet Assoc* 102 (8): 1145–55.

Dansinger, M. L., J. A. Gleason, J. L. Griffith, H. P. Selker, and E. J. Schaefer. 2005. "Comparison of the Atkins, Ornish, Weight Watchers, and Zone Diets for Weight Loss and Heart Disease Risk Reduction: A Randomized Trial." *JAMA* 293 (1): 43–53.

Davison, K. K., and L. L. Birch. 2002. "Obesigenic Families: Parents' Physical Activity and Dietary Intake Patterns Predict Girls' Risk of Overweight." *Int J Obes Relat Metab Disord* 26 (9): 1186–93.

Davison, K. K., T. M. Cutting, and L. L. Birch. 2003. "Parents' Activity-Related Parenting Practices Predict Girls' Physical Activity." *Med Sci Sports Exerc* 35 (9): 1589–95.

Dietz, W. H., and S. L. Gortmaker. 2001. "Preventing Obesity in Children and Adolescents." *Annu Rev Public Health* 22: 337–53.

Douglass, J. M., A. B. Douglass, and H. J. Silk. 2004. "A Practical Guide to Infant Oral Health." *Am Fam Physician* 70 (11): 2113–20.

Duyff, R. L. 1996. *American Dietetic Association Complete Food and Nutrition Guide.* Minneapolis: Chronimed Publishing.

Edelstein, B. L., and C. W. Douglass. 1995. "Dispelling the Myth That 50 Percent of U.S. Schoolchildren Have Never Had a Cavity." *Public Health Rep* 110 (5): 522–30; discussion 521, 531–33.

Eisenmann. J. C., R. T. Bartee, and M. Q. Wang. 2002. "Physical Activity, TV Viewing, and Weight in U.S. Youth: 1999 Youth Risk Behavior Survey." *Obes Res* 10 (5): 379–85.

Epstein, L. H., B. E. Saelens, and J. G. O'Brien. 1995. "Effects of Reinforcing Increases in Active Behavior Versus Decreases in Sedentary Behavior for Obese Children." *Int J Behav Med* 2 (1): 41–50.

ExRx.Net, LLC. "Colorful Choices: Fruit & Vegetable Color Codes." www.exrx.net/Nutrition/ColorCodes.html.

Faigenbaum, A. D. April–June 2001. "Physical Activity for Youth: Tips for Keeping Kids Healthy and Fit." *American College of Sports Medicine* 3–4.

Field, A. E., C. A. Camargo Jr., C. B. Taylor, C. S. Berkey, S. B. Roberts, and G. A. Colditz. 2001. "Peer, Parent, and Media Influences on the Development of Weight Concerns and Frequent Dieting Among Preadolescent and Adolescent Girls and Boys." *Pediatrics* 107 (1): 54–60.

Fontaine, K. R., D. T. Redden, C. Wang, A. O. Westfall, D. B. Allison. 2003. "Years of Life Lost Due to Obesity." *JAMA* 289: 187.

Food and Drug Administration. "How to Understand and Use the Nutrition Facts Label." www.cfsan.fda.gov/~acrobat/foodlab.pdf.

Francis, L. A., and L. L. Birch. 2005. "Maternal Influences on Daughters' Restrained Eating Behavior." *Health Psychol* 24 (6): 548–54.

———. 2006. "Does Eating During Television Viewing Affect Preschool Children's Intake?" *J Am Diet Assoc* 106 (4): 598–600.

Francis, L. A., Y. Lee, and L. L. Birch. 2003. "Parental Weight Status and Girls' Television Viewing, Snacking, and Body Mass Indexes." *Obes Res* 11 (1): 143–51.

"From Baby Bottle to Cup: Choose Training Cups Carefully, Use Them Temporarily." 2004. *J Am Dent Assoc* 135 (3): 387.

Fulkerson, J. A., D. Neumark-Sztainer, and M. Story. 2006. "Adolescent and Parent Views of Family Meals." *J Am Diet Assoc* 106 (4): 526–32.

Furuno, S., K. A. O'Reilly, C. M. Hosaka, T. Inatsuka, T. Allman, and B. Zeisloft. 1985. *Hawaii Early Learning Profile (HELP)*. Palo Alto, CA: VORT Corp.

Galloway, A. T., L. M. Fiorito, L. A. Francis, and L. L. Birch. 2006. "'Finish Your Soup': Counterproductive Effects of Pressuring Children to Eat on Intake and Affect." *Appetite* 46 (3): 318–23.

Gartner, L. M., J. Morton, R. A. Lawrence, A. J. Naylor, D. O'Hare, R. J. Schanler, and A. I. Eidelman. 2005. "Breastfeeding and the Use of Human Milk." *Pediatrics* 115 (2): 496–506.

Gatorade Sports Science Institute. "Beverage Comparison Chart." www.gssiweb-de .com/pdf/gatorade_bev_chart.pdf.

Gillman, M. W., S. L. Rifas-Shiman, A. L. Frazier, H. R. Rockett, C. A. Camargo Jr., A. E. Field, C. S. Berkey, and G. A. Colditz. 2000. "Family Dinner and Diet Quality Among Older Children and Adolescents." *Arch Fam Med* 9 (3): 235–40.

Glanz, Karen, Barbara K. Rimer, and Frances Marcus Lewis. 2002. *Health Behavior and Health Education: Theory, Research, and Practice*. San Francisco: Jossey-Bass.

Gonzalez, A. J., E. White, A. Kristal, and A. J. Littman. 2006. "Calcium Intake and 10-Year Weight Change in Middle-Aged Adults." *J Am Diet Assoc* 106 (7): 1066–73; quiz 1082.

Grunbaum, J. A., L. Kann, S. Kinchen, J. Ross, J. Hawkins, R. Lowry, W. A. Harris, T. McManus, D. Chyen, and J. Collins. 2004. "Youth Risk Behavior Surveillance— United States, 2003." *MMWR Surveill Summ* 53 (2): 1–96.

Halford, J. C., J. Gillespie, V. Brown, E. E. Pontin, and T. M. Dovey. 2004. "Effect of Television Advertisements for Foods on Food Consumption in Children." *Appetite* 42 (2): 221–25.

"Head Start Performance Standards." 2006. www.acf.hhs.gov/programs/hsb/perfor-mance/index.

Heber, D. 2002. *What Color Is Your Diet?* New York: Harper.

Hediger, M. L., M. D. Overpeck, R. J. Kuczmarski, and W. J. Ruan. 2001. "Association Between Infant Breastfeeding and Overweight in Young Children." *JAMA* 285 (19): 2453–60.

Helmrath, M. A., T. H. Inge, M. L. Brandt, and V. Garcia. 2006. *Scientific Principles and Practices: Pediatric Obesity, Surgery of Infants and Children*. 2nd ed. Philadelphia: Lippincott/Raven.

Hurst, N. M. 1988. *Breastfeeding Your Hospitalized Baby*. Edited by A. Myatt and B. Bartman. Houston: Texas Children's Hospital.

Institute of Medicine. "Food Marketing and the Diets of Children and Youth." 2005. www.iom.edu/kidsfoodmarketing.

Jago, R., M. L. Jonker, M. Missaghian, and T. Baranowski. 2006. "Effect of 4 Weeks of Pilates on the Body Composition of Young Girls." *Prev Med* 42 (3): 177–80.

Johnson, S. L., and L. L. Birch. 1994. "Parents' and Children's Adiposity and Eating Style." *Pediatrics* 94 (5): 653–61.

Keery, H., K. Boutelle, P. van den Berg, and J. K. Thompson. 2005. "The Impact of Appearance-Related Teasing by Family Members." *J Adolesc Health* 37 (2): 120–27.

Kirk, T. R. 2000. "Role of Dietary Carbohydrate and Frequent Eating in Body-Weight Control." *Proc Nutr Soc* 59 (3): 349–58.

Kleiman, R. E. 2004. *Pediatric Nutrition Handbook.* 5th ed. Elk Grove Village, IL: American Academy of Pediatrics.

Kosharek, Sharon M. 2003. *If Your Child Is Overweight: A Guide for Parents.* 2nd ed. Chicago: American Dietetic Association.

Kraut, A., S. Melamed, D. Gofer, and P. Froom. 2003. "Effect of School Age Sports on Leisure Time Physical Activity in Adults: The CORDIS Study." *Med Sci Sports Exerc* 35 (12): 2038–42.

Ludwig, D. S., C. B. Ebbeling, K. E. Peterson, and S. L. Gortmaker. 2004. "Hard Facts About Soft Drinks." *Arch Pediatr Adolesc Med* 158 (3): 290.

Maloney, M. J., J. McGuire, S. R. Daniels, and B. Specker. 1989. "Dieting Behavior and Eating Attitudes in Children." *Pediatrics* 84 (3): 482–89.

Matheson, D. M., J. D. Killen, Y. Wang, A. Varady, and T. N. Robinson. 2004. "Children's Food Consumption During Television Viewing." *Am J Clin Nutr* 79 (6): 1088–94.

Mitchell, M., and R. McKethan. Spring 2003. "Working with Overzealous Parents in a Youth Sport Setting." *Fit Society,* American College of Sports Medicine. www.acsm.org.

Moore, L. L., D. A. Lombardi, M. J. White, J. L. Campbell, S. A. Oliveria, and R. C. Ellison. 1991. "Influence of Parents' Physical Activity Levels on Activity Levels of Young Children." *J Pediatr* 118 (2): 215–19.

National Center for Chronic Disease Prevention, National Health and Nutrition Examination Survey. "CDC Growth Charts." 2000. www.cdc.gov/growthcharts/.

National Center for Health Statistics in collaboration with National Center for Chronic Disease Prevention and Health Promotion. "Clinical Growth Charts." 2000. www.cdc.gov/growthcharts.

Nelson, J. A., K. Carpenter, and M. A. Chiasson. 2006. "Diet, Activity, and Overweight Among Preschool-Age Children Enrolled in the Special Supplemental Nutrition Program for Women, Infants, and Children (WIC)." *Prev Chronic Dis* 3 (2): A49.

Nemours Foundation. "Learning About Fats." 2004. www.kidshealth.org/kid/stay_healthy/food/fat.html.

Newman, Jack. "What Is Colostrum? How Does It Benefit My Baby?" 2006. www.lalecheleague.org/FAQ/colostrum.

Nicklas, T., and R. Johnson. 2004. "Position of the American Dietetic Association: Dietary Guidance for Healthy Children Ages 2 to 11 Years." *J Am Diet Assoc* 104 (4): 660–77.

Nicklas, T. A., C. E. O'Neil, and G. S. Berenson. 1998. "Nutrient Contribution of Breakfast, Secular Trends, and the Role of Ready-to-Eat Cereals: A Review of Data from the Bogalusa Heart Study." *Am J Clin Nutr* 67 (4): 757S–63S.

Nicklas, T. A., S. J. Yang, T. Baranowski, I. Zakeri, and G. Berenson. 2003. "Eating Patterns and Obesity in Children: The Bogalusa Heart Study." *Am J Prev Med* 25 (1): 9–16.

Orlet Fisher, J., B. J. Rolls, and L. L. Birch. 2003. "Children's Bite Size and Intake of an Entree Are Greater with Large Portions than with Age-Appropriate or Self-Selected Portions." *Am J Clin Nutr* 77 (5): 1164–70.

Ortega, R. M., A. M. Requejo, A. M. Lopez-Sobaler, M. E. Quintas, P. Andres, M. R. Redondo, B. Navia, M. D. Lopez-Bonilla, and T. Rivas. 1998. "Difference in the Breakfast Habits of Overweight/Obese and Normal Weight Schoolchildren." *Int J Vitam Nutr Res* 68 (2): 125–32.

Owen, C. G., R. M. Martin, P. H. Whincup, G. D. Smith, and D. G. Cook. 2005. "Effect of Infant Feeding on the Risk of Obesity Across the Life Course: A Quantitative Review of Published Evidence." *Pediatrics* 115 (5): 1367–77.

Parsons, T. J., C. Power, and O. Manor. 2001. "Fetal and Early Life Growth and Body Mass Index from Birth to Early Adulthood in 1958 British Cohort: Longitudinal Study." *BMJ* 323 (7325): 1331–35.

Pate, R. R., G. W. Heath, M. Dowda, and S. G. Trost. 1996. "Associations Between Physical Activity and Other Health Behaviors in a Representative Sample of US Adolescents." *Am J Public Health* 86 (11): 1577–81.

"Position of the American Dietetic Association: Benchmarks for Nutrition Programs in Child Care Settings." 2005. *J Am Diet Assoc* 105 (6): 979–86.

"Position of the American Dietetic Association: Individual-, Family-, School-, and Community-Based Interventions for Pediatric Overweight." 2006. *J Am Diet Assoc* 106 (6): 925–45.

Preboth, M. 2002. "Physical Activity in Infants, Toddlers, and Preschoolers." *Am Fam Physician* 65 (8): 1694.

Reilly, J. J., J. Armstrong, A. R. Dorosty, P. M. Emmett, A. Ness, I. Rogers, C. Steer, and A. Sherriff. 2005. "Early Life Risk Factors for Obesity in Childhood: Cohort Study." *BMJ* 330 (7504): 1357.

Resnick, M. D., P. S. Bearman, R. W. Blum, K. E. Bauman, K. M. Harris, J. Jones, J. Tabor, T. Beuhring, R. E. Sieving, M. Shew, M. Ireland, L. H. Bearinger, and J. R. Udry. 1997. "Protecting Adolescents from Harm: Findings from the National Longitudinal Study on Adolescent Health." *JAMA* 278 (10): 823–32.

Rising, R., and F. Lifshitz. 2005. "Relationship Between Maternal Obesity and Infant Feeding Interactions." *Nutr J* 4:17.

Rolls, B. J., and Robert Barnett. 2000. *Volumetrics: Feel Full on Fewer Calories*. New York: Harper.

Satter, Ellyn. 1987. *How to Get Your Kid to Eat . . . but Not Too Much*. Palo Alto, CA: Bull Publishing.

———. 2000. *Child of Mine: Feeding with Love and Good Sense*. 3rd ed. Palo Alto, CA: Bull Publishing.

Sayer, A. A., H. E. Syddall, E. M. Dennison, H. J. Gilbody, S. L. Duggleby, C. Cooper, D. J. Barker, and D. I. Phillips. 2004. "Birth Weight, Weight at 1 y of Age, and Body Composition in Older Men: Findings from the Hertfordshire Cohort Study." *Am J Clin Nutr* 80 (1): 199–203.

Schaefer-Graf, U. M., J. Pawliczak, D. Passow, R. Hartmann, R. Rossi, C. Buhrer, T. Harder, A. Plagemann, K. Vetter, and O. Kordonouri. 2005. "Birth Weight and Parental BMI Predict Overweight in Children from Mothers with Gestational Diabetes." *Diabetes Care* 28 (7): 1745–50.

Schwimmer, J. B., T. M. Burwinkle, and J. W. Varni. "Health-Related Quality of Life of Severely Obese Children and Adolescents." 2003. *JAMA* 289 14: 1813-19.

"School Health Policies and Programs Study (SHPPS) 2000: A Summary Report." 2001. *J Sch Health* 71 (7): 251–350.

Siega-Riz, A. M., T. Carson, and B. Popkin. 1998. "Three Squares or Mostly Snacks—What Do Teens Really Eat? A Sociodemographic Study of Meal Patterns." *J Adolesc Health* 22 (1): 29–36.

Siega-Riz, A. M., B. M. Popkin, and T. Carson. 1998. "Trends in Breakfast Consumption for Children in the United States from 1965–1991." *Am J Clin Nutr* 67 (4): 748S–56S.

Simon, G. E., M. Von Korff, K. Saunders, D. L. Miglioretti, P. K. Crane, G. van Belle, and R. C. Kessler. 2006. "Association Between Obesity and Psychiatric Disorders in the US Adult Population." *Arch Gen Psychiatry* 63 (7): 824–30.

Sothern, J., N. Udall Jr., R. M. Suskind, A. Vargas, and U. Blecker. 2000. "Weight Loss and Growth Velocity in Obese Children After Very Low Calorie Diet, Exercise, and Behavior Modification." *Acta Paediatr* 89 (9): 1036–43.

Stang, J. 2006. "Improving the Eating Patterns of Infants and Toddlers." *J Am Diet Assoc* 106 (1 Suppl 1): S7–9.

Story, M., K. Holt, and D. Sofka, eds. 2002. *Bright Futures in Practice: Nutrition.* 2nd ed. Arlington, VA: National Center for Education in Maternal and Child Health.

Strauss, R. S., and J. Knight. 1999. "Influence of the Home Environment on the Development of Obesity in Children." *Pediatrics* 103 (6): e85.

Texas Children's Hospital. 2005. *Pediatric Nutrition Reference Guide.* 7th ed. Houston: TCH.

Tudor-Locke, C., R. P. Pangrazi, C. B. Corbin, W. J. Rutherford, S. D. Vincent, A. Raustorp, L. M. Tomson, and T. F. Cuddihy. 2004. "BMI-Referenced Standards for Recommended Pedometer-Determined Steps/Day in Children." *Prev Med* 38 (6): 857–64.

University of Washington, News & Information Services. 2002. "I'll Drink to That." *University Week,* April 11.

U.S. Council of Economic Advisers. 2000. "Teens and Their Parents in the 21st Century: An Examination of Trends in Teen Behavior and the Role of Parental Involvement." clinton3.nara.gov/WH/EOP/CEA/html/Teens_Paper_Final.pdf.

———. "My Pyramid: Eat Right. Exercise. Have Fun." www.teamnutrition.usda.gov/Resources/mpk_poster.pdf.

———. "Meal Patterns: Child and Adult Care Food Program." www.fns.usda.gov/cnd/Care/ProgramBasics/Meals/Meal_Patterns.

U.S. Department of Health and Human Services. 1996. "Physical Activity and Health: A Report of the Surgeon General." Atlanta: Centers for Disease Control and Prevention and National Center for Chronic Disease Prevention and Health Promotion.

———. 2001. "The Surgeon General's Call to Action to Prevent and Decrease Overweight and Obesity." Rockville, MD: U.S. Department of Health and Human Services, Public Health Service, and Office of the Surgeon General.

———. "Dietary Guidelines for Americans." 2005. www.healthierus.gov/dietary guidelines/.

———. "Overweight and Obesity: Health Consequences." www.surgeongeneral.gov/topics/obesity/calltoaction/fact_consequences.htm.

Weiss, R., J. Dziura. T. S. Burgert, W. V. Tamborlane, S. E. Taksali, C. W. Yeckel, K. Allen, M. Lopes, M. Savoye, J. Morrison, R. S. Sherwin, and S. Caprio. 2004. "Obesity and the Metabolic Syndrome in Children and Adolescents," *N Engl J Med* 350 (23) 2362–74.

Whitaker, R. C. 2004. "Predicting Preschooler Obesity at Birth: The Role of Maternal Obesity in Early Pregnancy." *Pediatrics* 114 (1): e29–36.

About the Authors and Contributors

Patricia Ahern, R.D., C.S.P., L.D., coauthor on "Setting Good Habits with the Pre-K Set," is a senior clinical pediatric dietitian and a certified specialist in pediatric nutrition at Texas Children's Hospital.

Roberta Anding, M.S., R.D., C.S.S.D., L.D., C.D.E., coauthor on "Older Teens: Teaching Without Telling," "When Your Child Needs an Expert," and general editor, is a clinical dietitian and certified diabetes educator in the Department of Pediatrics, Adolescent and Sports Medicine, at Baylor College of Medicine.

Dawn Bunting, R.D., C.S.P., L.D., general editor, is assistant director of Clinical Nutrition Services and a certified specialist in pediatric nutrition in the Department of Food and Nutrition Services at Texas Children's Hospital.

Lavonne Carlson, coauthor of "Creating Change" and general editor.

Claudia Conkin, M.S., R.D., L.D., general editor, is director of Food and Nutrition Services at Texas Children's Hospital.

Stephen Habetz, M.S.P.T., M.H.A., coauthor of "Making Fitness Fun and Effective," is a physical therapist and manager in the Department of Physical Medicine and Rehabilitation at Texas Children's Hospital.

Albert Hergenroeder, M.D., general editor and coauthor on teens, is the chief of Texas Children's Adolescent Medicine Service and Clinic, Sports Medicine Clinic, and Young Women's Clinic, professor of pediatrics, and head of Adolescent Medicine and Sports Medicine at Baylor College of Medicine.

Heather Holden, M.Ed., R.D., L.D., C.D.E., coauthor of "Smart Behaviors to Start Slimming Down," is a research dietitian/exercise physiologist and certified diabetes educator in the Department of Pediatrics, Endocrinology, and Metabolism at Baylor College of Medicine.

Marisa Juarez-Congelosi, M.P.H., R.D., L.D., coauthor of "Smart Behaviors to Start Slimming Down," is a clinical dietitian in the Department of Food and Nutrition Services at Texas Children's Hospital.

Lauren Kelley, M.S., R.D., L.D., C.P.T., coauthor on "Staying Tuned to Tweens" and "Older Teens: Teaching Without Telling," is a clinical dietitian in the Department of Pediatrics, Adolescent and Sports Medicine at Baylor College of Medicine.

Kristi L. King, M.P.H., R.D., L.D., coauthor on "Healthy Food Choices," is a clinical dietitian in the Department of Gastroenterology, Hepatology, and Nutrition at Texas Children's Hospital.

William J. Klish, M.D., in the Department of Gastroenterology, Hepatology, and Nutrition at Texas Children's Hospital and professor of pediatrics at Baylor College of Medicine, is a general editor and contributor to the book. He is a founding member of the Coalition for a Healthy and Active America and currently chairs the Texas Department of Health Obesity Task Force.

Kristi Ludwig, M.S., R.D., L.D., coauthor on "Staying Tuned to Tweens," is a clinical dietitian in the Department of Food and Nutrition Services at Texas Children's Hospital.

Shelly McBride, M.S., R.D., L.D., coauthor on "Healthy Food Choices," is a clinical dietitian in the Department of Food and Nutrition Services at Texas Children's Hospital.

Cindy Mogannam, M.P.H., R.D., L.D., coauthor on "Setting Good Habits with the Pre-K Set," is a clinical dietitian in the Department of Food and Nutrition Services at Texas Children's Hospital.

Sarah Phillips, M.S., R.D., L.D., coauthor on "Creating Change: The ROAD to Success" and general editor, is manager of Nutrition Support in Department of Gastroenterology, Hepatology, and Nutrition at Texas Children's Hospital.

Lisa Symeonidis, M.P.H., R.D., C.S.P., L.D., author of "Action Is Everything in Grade School," is a clinical dietitian in the Department of Food and Nutrition Services at Texas Children's Hospital.

Daniela Torres Marco, M.S., R.D., L.D., I.B.C.L.C., author on "From the Beginning: Feeding Your Infant," is a lactation specialist and clinical dietitian in the department of Food and Nutrition Services at Texas Children's Hospital.

Susanne Trout, R.D., L.D., I.B.C.L.C., R.L.C., coauthor of "When Your Child Needs an Expert," is certified in childhood and adolescent weight management and is the clinical dietitian for bariatric surgery at Texas Children's Hospital in the Department of Food and Nutrition Services.

Terry Whaley, M.P.H., R.D., L.D., coauthor on "Healthy Food Choices," is Assistant Director of Patient Services, Food and Nutrition Services at Texas Children's Hospital.

Katy Wilkinson, P.T., coauthor of "Making Fitness Fun and Effective," is a physical therapist and manager in Physical Medicine and Rehabilitation at Texas Children's Hospital.

Contributors

Carmen Mikhail, Ph.D., provided expertise on behavioral topics throughout the book, is a psychologist in the Eating Disorders Clinic at Texas Children's Hospital.

Maureen E. Carroll, L.C.S.W., provided expertise on behavioral topics throughout the book, is a behavioral therapist for the Eating Disorders Clinic at Texas Children's Hospital.

Christina Kontos, L.C.S.W., provided expertise on behavioral topics, is a behavioral therapist for the Eating Disorders Clinic at Texas Children's Hospital.

Index

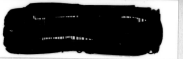